To Ellen

wishing you health
and happiness!

love and blessing
Dr Natalya

HEALTH AND WELLNESS

for

BUSY WOMEN

A Guide to Balance, Heal and Transform Your Life

By Natalya Fazylova, DNP

Health and Wellness for Busy Women: A Guide to Balance, Heal and Transform Your Life
First Edition

IMPORTANT NOTE:
The content provided in this book is for general instruction only. Each person's physical, emotional, and spiritual condition is unique. The instruction in this book is not intended to replace or interrupt the reader's relationship with a health care professional. Please consult your health care practitioner for matters pertaining to your specific health and diet concerns. The author and editors are not responsible for any specific health or allergy needs that may require medical supervision, and are not liable for any damage or negative consequences from any treatment, action, application or preparation, to any person reading or following the information in this book. References are provided for informational purposes only and do not constitute endorsement of any websites or other sources.

Every effort has been made to make this book as complete and accurate as possible. However, there may be mistakes, both typographical and in content. Therefore, this should be only used as a guide, not as an ultimate source of information. Furthermore, this book contains information that is current only up to the printing date, websites listed may change.

ISBN : 978-0692434215
LCCN: 2015920979
Printed in the United States of America
Library of Congress Cataloging in Publication Data

Editors: Nancy Iankowitz and Mary Dvorak
Illustrator: Andrea Small
Interior design: Maggie Pagratis
Cover design: Julia Lin

Dedicated with gratitude and love to my grandmother
whose final advice to me was:
"You only have one life to live-live it to the fullest."

CONTENTS

PART III

HEALING YOUR SOUL

PART IV

SELF-TRANSFORMATION

Acknowledgements

I would like to extend my sincerest thanks and acknowledge the following people for their unique contribution to this book:

My wonderful and dedicated editors Dr. Nancy Iankowitz and Marie Dvorak, who's skillful, knowledgeable and sensitive editing brought emphasis and clarity to my words and thoughts.

The contributors: Andrea Beaman, Kelly Ahearn, Dr Hyla Cass, Dr. Dana Cohen, Ellen Gavrielov, Svetlana Kotlovskiy, Dr. Nancy Iankowitz, Dr. Ronald Hoffman, Dr. Arkady Lipnitsky, Marcin Michula, Inna Natkovitch, Dr. Daniel Roshan and Dr. Jacob Teitelbaum who worked diligently to provide up-to-date information in their specialty areas and were patient with many requests that were always quickly addressed.

My talented illustrator-Andrea Small for her beautiful and creative pictures.

My talented and aspiring cover artist Julia Lin for her colorful book cover that expertly evokes anticipation to read this book.

My amazing and courageous friend and colleague Margarita Israilova who have supported me through this process acting as a facilitator, sounding board and advisor.

My beloved family: my husband Mishoel, and my sons Moisey and Daniel for support, understanding, insightful comments and suggestions.

Lastly, but most importantly I acknowledge with love and gratitude my wonderful friends and family for constant support and encouragement through this process.

Introduction

Welcome to the Busy Women's Guide to Health and Wellness

Hello Busy Ladies: This book is for YOU!

Working moms, who balance multitasking with your work, family, partner, children, parents and in-laws, when was the last time you felt guilt-free about something great you did for yourself?

Stay-at-home moms, busy with raising children, making your home a loving and comfortable place as you cook, clean, grocery shop, and drive to and from soccer practice and ballet lessons, this is for those of you who are the foundation and glue for your family and household, putting yourselves last in order to keep everything running smoothly. When was the last time you were validated with a heartfelt, "What would we/I do without you?" Is it easier to recall the last time you heard, "What do you DO all day?" What you do is invest in the future of the world, well aware that the time, effort, and energy it takes to raise children is exactly that. Children are our future. Did you ever consider that you might be responsible for raising a future scientist, a famous composer, or even a future president of this country? It is important to invest in yourself, and this book is an opportunity for you to find time to do just that.

Sisters, daughters, wives, and life partners, busy acquiring degrees, working on establishing your careers, doing research, becoming part of life's landscape in countless ways, including but not limited to caring for aging parents, and volunteering time, energy, and effort as unsung heroes of society. It is not an easy task to find time for yourself while facing constant deadlines as you juggle projects and meetings.

Regardless of where you are in your life right now, we all get buried in the endless details of work or everyday living. For those who want to live a happier, healthier, and more peaceful life but get so busy with mundane matters, believing you don't have time or energy to invest in yourself and fearing you can't add one more thing to your already crammed schedule. . . this book is for YOU.

When I started writing this book, I didn't know what format it should take. Should it be 6 weeks to healing and transformation? But then I thought, there are so many excellent books already written. I personally read several of them and enjoyed them immensely; however, when I tried to accomplish everything in 6 or 8 weeks as was suggested in the book, it didn't happen. Something always came up. Something will *always* come up – whether it be a deadline at work, children getting sick, or some other family emergency to take precedence over all our best intentions. The bottom line is that life happens and can flush all our efforts down the drain until we master the art of taking charge of our own well-being.

Then I considered writing a self-help book but soon realized authors of such books often come across as "Ms. /Mr. Perfect with all the answers," leaving readers with a feeling of self-dissatisfaction. My goal with this book is to share my personal search for and discovery of interventions that improved my own health and enriched my family lifestyle, with the clear understanding that change is difficult. Change takes time and energy. It requires knowledge and understanding regarding why one needs to heal and transform. It takes personal commitment and motivation. So in this book, I decided to share evidence-based knowledge about what health is and why it is important to pursue a healthy lifestyle.

The human body is built to self-repair. We see this as evidenced by a healing cut on a finger or scraped knee. The body heals when permitted to. Sickness and degenerative diseases are not part of aging; rather, they are strongly influenced by poor lifestyle and eating habits. It is my hope that with the information provided by this book, readers will recognize that health and vitality are within reach and fulfillment of personal health is in their hands. The lifelong adventure to healing and transformation is a rewarding one requiring effort and dedication.

With one step at a time, each person determines a personal pace. Each day has its challenges and rewards. I can promise that with honest desire and a heartfelt effort to achieve short and long-term goals, success will be yours. This book helps with each step. Some readers will begin to see results within 3 months; others may take longer. Whatever your pace, you will get where you want to be one step at a time, and it is all "okay" since your life is yours and yours alone. My hope is that this book facilitates a beautiful beginning to your lifelong journey of healing and transformation. I hope your Flower of Life blossoms with new vibrant, energetic colors of vitality.

To your health, healing, and transformation.

HOW TO USE THIS BOOK

The Roman poet Virgil, who lived in 30 BC, once said, "The greatest wealth is health." In this one sentence, he captured the whole essence of our life and well-being. When healthy, it takes minimal effort and just a bit of persistence to achieve our goals. Unfortunately, when we are sick, all the wealth in the world may not be able to bring our health back.

The Dalai Lama once said, *"Man surprised me most about humanity. Because he sacrifices his health in order to make money. Then he sacrifices money to recuperate his health. And then he is so anxious about the future that he does not enjoy the present; the result being that he does not live in the present or the future; he lives as if he is never going to die, and then dies having never really lived."*

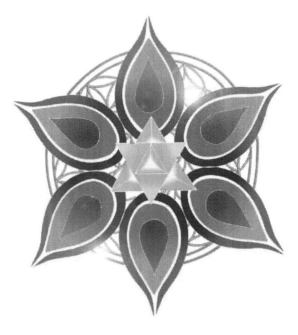

Merkaba — Flower of Life

While working on this book, I came across a Merkaba sign — the Flower of Life (FOL), a universal symbol said to contain all the patterns of creation. This geometric design is associated with the most ancient cultures and has been found in many countries, including Egypt (the oldest known), Turkey, Italy, Masada Israel, Mount Sinai, Austria, Denmark, Bulgaria, India, Spain, Japan, and China. The Merkaba is symbolic of the human body encompassed by life energy that is directed for the well-being of the person using the Merkaba, thereby protecting and healing the person. This symbol is considered more than just lucky; it is said to help us connect with our soul and feel healthy, scientifically as well as holistically. The six circles of the flower—or six points of a star, similar to the Star of David—represent two overlapping triangles and the reconciliation of opposites: male and female, fire and water, and so on. Their combination symbolizes unity and harmony.

When I read the definition of the Merkaba FOL sign, a thought crystallized in my mind that it would be a perfect symbol of healing for this book. We women are the beginning of a new life, with an inner ability to heal and protect people around us. We strive for unity, harmony, and peace. Unfortunately, all too often, we are so busy healing and protecting everything and everybody around us that we forget about ourselves. The Flower of Life symbol with its six dimensions of healing is your guide throughout this book. There are 6 interconnected dimensions to health and healing:

1. Mind
2. Body
3. Soul
4. Environment
5. Lifestyle
6. Relationship

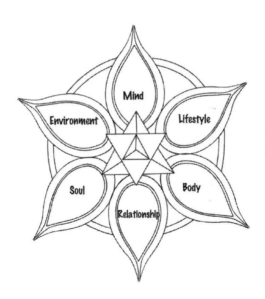

Healing Flower of Life

To lead a healthy and a happy life, all of these six dimensions should be in balance. In this book, I will discuss all six dimensions in greater detail within four separate sections.

In Part One, we will discuss the mind and body connection; how to calm your mind to achieve optimal wellness.

In Part Two, we will cover things you need to know in order to help heal your body. We will talk about the hormonal balances, diet, exercise, sleep, and beauty routine needed for your specific body type.

In Part Three, we will talk about the importance of taking care of your soul. We will cover topics of self-love, self-esteem, self-value, as well as relationships and living your life purposefully.

In Part Four, we will use all the information you learned in the first three parts to help you start your journey to transformation. Thomas Jefferson said, *"If you want something you've never had, you must be willing to do something you've never done before."* This is what this guide is all about. It will enable you to open your mind to new horizons and help you change your behavior so you may begin healing and transforming yourself in order to live the life you deserve.

PART I

HEALING THE MIND

Chapter 1

CALMING YOUR MIND

"If an individual has a calm state of mind, that person's attitudes and views will be calm and tranquil even in the presence of great agitation."
Tensin Gyatso, the 14th Dalai Lama

If you are a busy woman familiar with multitasking; solving problems; taking care of family, children, and loved ones; conquering new challenges and opportunities at work or school; and accomplishing myriad things, your mind probably races with ideas while thoughts trip over one another, often keeping both your mind and life in utter turmoil. You may find there is never enough time to set aside moments to breathe in the "simple things." You are so busy rushing through the present moment you often neglect internal balance. How can you stay balanced when all that swirls around you demands your attention every second?

If you could take a few minutes to help your busy mind stop spinning in a seemingly endless circuit of worry, fear, deadlines, and tasks, the inevitable negativity would dissolve into a vision of internal peace. Your life situation might remain unchanged, but your perception would facilitate a healthful outlook. This state is where the healing of your mind begins.

When your mind is calm, and you feel centered and balanced, you actually become more efficient. Daily challenges become easier to conquer. Your focus sharpens, and you become more open and able to spread your love while accepting it from others.

When your mind is calm, your inside world is at peace. You become more able to hear and understand messages from your soul and your body. Your body is greatly influenced by your mind, and there is a very strong connection between your mind, your body, and your health. In this book, we will be discussing in detail how your lifestyle, including the food you eat, number of hours you sleep, and the exercise you do, affects your health.

We will outline easy and doable regimens to transform your life with a healthier you. In this section, I will begin by addressing the mind/body connections that have a tremendous influence on your health. While changing your diet and lifestyle may help achieve certain positive results, healing and calming your mind requires special consideration.

Your mind is very powerful. It influences everything you do and your perception of everything that happens in your life. There is a saying—*change your way of thinking if you want to change your way of life*. It is very important to understand your mind in order to change your mindset, which must occur in order to grow and improve your lifestyle.

This book offers a wealth of information on how to achieve a healthier lifestyle; however, if your mindset is not changed, it indicates you are not yet ready to become successful in this effort at this time. That is okay. Honest self-reflection helps us identify what might be in our way and why we hold on to certain patterns of behavior. Once we identify our unhealthy mindset and the reasons for it, the journey to improve it can begin again. My goal for this book is to help you understand yourself and your mind, help you to find your inner self that defines you, and help you to change your mind set to achieve peace and balance in your life. Let's get started and learn how to calm your mind first.

Pearls of Wisdom from My Grandmother

When I was a child, I spent a lot of time with my grandmother, who helped raise me. She was an exceptional woman, with a big heart and warm smile, who was generous with her love. She was an incredible woman, who raised nine children while working as an accountant at a school and managing a farm. She was a supremely awesome woman, full of wisdom and advice that I learned to heed.

Her conversations were filled with references to the Torah and ancient proverbs and wisdom; she would share these living principles with me, saying, "There is an old saying regarding this topic...." She taught me life lessons throughout my childhood, some of which I could not understand or appreciate at the time; they became more meaningful as I moved on with my life and had to face and deal with my own life challenges. On the pages that follow, I would like to share with you her pearls of wisdom that taught me life lessons that are still guiding me through my life journey.

Take Time to Calm Your Mind

It was a day before Passover eve. I was visiting my grandmother who was busy with preparations for a holiday dinner that our whole family was gathered for and would celebrate. As you could imagine, the house was in an uproar with delicious varieties of dishes and pastries being prepared, rooms being aired out and cleaned, and a splendid table being set with very special holiday dinnerware. We had all assembled to help. My sister, mother, cousins, and aunts were all there to lend a hand.

Soon we became full of the traditional holiday frustration that was the result of too much to do and too little time to accomplish all that needed to be done. At a strategic point during this particular experience, my grandmother asked us all to stop working to take a few minutes to sit down because she wanted to tell us a story. We were all surprised since there was so much to do. We were already tired, and guests would be arriving soon.

We asked her if she could tell her story while we continued working. The answer as you probably guessed was "no." She offered us a cup of tea and then shared the story about the wood cutter and his ax—which you've probably heard before, but in case you didn't or need a reminder, I'll summarize it here.

This story is about a woodcutter who busily cut his wood from sunrise to sundown. He worked hard every day. His effort was tremendous and consistent; however, the amount of wood he cut as the days progressed didn't reflect all the energy he was putting in. Instead of cutting greater quantities of lumber, he was cutting less and less until one of his neighbors stopped by to tell him to take a few minutes to sharpen his ax.

With this story, the message my grandmother conveyed was that no matter how busy and complicated life is, it is important to take a moment to calm yourself and your mind. Calming your mind helps you to use it to its full potential; giving your mind and body a few minutes of rest helps renew your energy so that you can perform more efficiently, become more creative, and be open to enrichment and learning. Sometimes we require more than just a few minutes, and we find it easier to follow a few hints along the way. Here are a few ideas that might help you to calm your mind and achieve inner peace.

Embrace Positivity and Stop Negativity

Is our glass half-full or half-empty? Staying positive *all* the time is not only difficult, it is unrealistic. The trick is in our attitude about what is going on around us—keeping perspective is key. Challenges that many of us face throughout our lives often make it trying for us to believe "everything is going to be fine," but there is a practical and very realistic way to appreciate the bright side, the silver lining around the dark clouds.

Upon examination, we realize that when we are faced with situations that are less than pleasant, it is often not the situation itself that causes us so much pain and suffering; rather, it is **our reaction** to the situation governed by our mindset that causes us to suffer. It is worthwhile to master the art of centering ourselves in the face of challenges. First we need to learn how to respond to situations with a positive attitude, calm demeanor, and peaceful mind.

A lot of major life crises that we face are often not as painful or hopeless as we believe them to be. Each challenge provides a learning opportunity for growth and development. Staying positive and optimistic doesn't mean that we keep our heads in the clouds or hide behind rose colored glasses; positive thinking doesn't mean that we are ignoring reality. Positive thinking means that we understand and embrace the reality of our life situation, but we are approaching it with a positive mindset and in a more productive way.

When you face a life crisis, ask yourself, "What is the worst thing that can happen in this scenario?" Take your concerns to their logical conclusion. Then ask yourself if there something you are able to do at this point in time to change the situation? Is it within your power to make it better? If so, how?

These questions help you to view the problem more objectively and rationally. It is essential to have this perspective when dealing with any challenge. Reminding yourself that the terrible situation might also have a positive outcome that you might actually benefit from is another possible result of this exercise in centering.

There are some women who seem to enjoy spending time feeling miserable about themselves. They tend to blame everything and everybody around them for whatever went wrong. The "victim" role we may tend to fall into is not healthy. If you find yourself complaining about being tired, make a healthy decision to take control and get more sleep or work meditation into your day. If you find yourself complaining about the inconvenience of having children, think about all the women who wished they could have children of their own, and feel grateful for your situation.

There is a quote about gratitude that is worth keeping in mind: "*I complained that I had no shoes until I met a man who had no feet.*" Gratitude goes a long way in helping us gain perspective. So the next time you complain that you have three daughters and no sons or that your husband watches television rather than helping with the kids, count your blessings that you have a family. When you feel stressed that your house is a mess, count your blessings that you have a roof over your head. If you don't have time for this or for that, **make** the time by prioritizing.

Another common error we women make is that we judge ourselves harshly. We believe if we don't do something perfectly or up to our own standards, we feel as if we failed. We are often unreasonably hard on ourselves. Congratulations on reading this far. It shows that you are interested in self-improvement and learning how to appreciate and balance your own mind, body and spirit. This means you will heal, and once healed; you can do more for others.

We begin to heal by recognizing our long list of potential misery and then making an active decision to not remain absorbed in it. Now it is time to decide to take control and gain perspective. This all starts with recognizing that we have the power to change our mindsets, stop being miserable, stop being negative, and learn to be positive and grateful for our lives.

I would like to offer a tip I find helpful—you can use it whenever you feel miserable and pitiful. Try reframing the stressful situation and then asking yourself, "***What could be better than this?***"

You might say something such as, "I am a mother of two beautiful, healthy children who are the joy of my life. ***What could be better than this?*** I have a great partner and a soul mate, who helps me to raise my children and has stayed by my side through all the difficult times. *What could be better than this*? I am strong and healthy, have an education and a job that I enjoy. *What could be better than this*? I have wonderful parents who helped to raise me and gave me the opportunity to receive my education. *What could be better than this*? This list could go on and on. I am sure we all have a lot of things in our life to be grateful for and be positive about. Positive thinking helps us deal with our lives in a more efficient and productive way.

Eliminate the Clutter - Stop Worrying

I'm guessing I'm not alone in having the following experience: after a busy day filled with tasks, I look forward to lying down in bed with the hopes of getting some rest or much needed sleep only to discover that my mind is unable to calm down and relax. Does your mind stay busy with trying to solve problems? Is your mind cluttered with overactive thoughts on different topics from the past or worries about the future? Do you relive long-since resolved confrontation(s) with another person, which are still very unpleasant to remember? Do you relive one or more problems in your past?

No matter how hard you think about it, worrying about the past will not change anything. Torturing yourself with guilty thoughts, such as "if only I'd done this" and "if I only I'd said that" will not help either. Thinking about the past without a plan for changing your behavior in the future is a waste of precious time.

Thoughts can be distracting or energizing. As stated, guilt, worry, and fear distract. Planning and reflecting can energize. Worry about the future is an example of self-distraction. I am not telling you to sit by, ignoring red flags while waiting for disasters to happen. I am a firm believer in prevention. But there is a difference between obsessing over "spilled milk" and observing the fact, cleaning it up, and preparing for the future to avoid the error next time.

For instance, when dealing with a situation you know is likely to repeat at some future time, try to analyze it to see if there is something you can do about it now to prevent repetition or any negative consequences. If it is out of your hands, and there is nothing that can be done, then let it be.

My grandmother had another good "***wisdom pearl***" I would like to share: *"Don't worry about the problem that you are not facing yet; you will have plenty of time to worry about it when the time comes."* Again, this is not to say we should not plan for the future. It cautions that borrowing trouble is not what we need to spend energy on.

As the Dalai Lama said, *"If a problem is fixable, if a situation is such that you can do something about it, then there is no need to worry. If it's not fixable, then there is no help in worrying. There is no benefit in worrying whatsoever."* So stop worrying, and clear the clutter from your mind. Stop regretting your past and fearing your future. Both of these activities cause you misery. Start enjoying your present.

Stop Controlling Everything

Busy women generally have an overwhelming urge to control everything and everybody in their life. You may have experienced a similar feeling. Have you ever been terrified of losing control of your circumstances because you think that if you lose control of things around you, you might then lose control over yourself? This is often expressed behaviorally by trying to control people in your life, such as your children and your spouse, to the point where they become so dependent on you, they might find it difficult or impossible to survive on their own. You may have convinced yourself that if you don't control them and their actions, disaster is inevitable.

Your wish to control them actually creates more problems and responsibilities for you and also gives you even more things to worry about. I had my own "wake-up" call and would like to share it with you now. Before I do, I'd like you to stop for a moment and think, "Do I really have to do it all? Do I really need to control everything and everybody in my life?"

Now, for my "wake-up" call: Two years ago, I had to attend a conference for three days in another city, and my family couldn't travel with me. I'd never left my husband and my children by themselves before, so I agonized for several days before departure. In my mind, I thought, "How are they going to manage without me? Will they have enough food to eat? Who is going to help my children with their homework?" While these are valuable and valid concerns for a loving, caring mother to have, obsessing over them is not healthy for anyone. I was obsessing.

I left the house on the day of my flight with a sinking feeling in my gut and images of a burned down house and starved family upon my return. I spent three days at the conference with my colleagues, worrying about situation at home. When I came back home expecting the worst, the house was still in its place, strong and sound. It was not burned down, and what is more, it was clean! My family didn't starve; they managed to cook some food for themselves or order take-out. I was relieved. Of course, not everything was done the way I do it, but it was done. I kept my mouth shut and was truly grateful that my family survived without me. I realized that by controlling everything around me, I wasn't giving my family an opportunity to live and experience their lives fully.

Children need to grow and learn; they need to make their own mistakes, experience their own success, and accept responsibility for their own decisions and life choices. Being a control freak is not only time-consuming and exhausting, but it is actually disruptive to a healthy growing process for yourself as well as for your family.

It is healthy and important to show your family that you have faith in them, that you trust they are strong and capable, and that you value yourself enough to pay attention to yourself. Have faith. Calm your mind by centering yourself as you find balance in your thoughts and reflections. Focus on positive things in your life; learn to trust yourself and the people around you. Everyone wins in this scenario.

Stress Management

Stress is inevitable in your life, and your psychological and emotional response to stress causes myriad changes in your body. These days, you could get exposed to stressful situations 40–50 times a day. Every negative thought, belief, and feeling forces your body to release stress hormones such as adrenaline and cortisol. These hormones switch your body's mechanism to "fight/flight" mode while simultaneously shutting down your body's self-repair mode. After the crisis, when your body relaxes, it gets into "self-repair" mode as it tries to heal and recover damaged parts. So when you think positive thoughts, laugh, and have positive feelings and beliefs, your body actually releases hormones and substances like dopamine, nitric oxide, and endorphins that help you to recover and heal yourself.

It is not how much stress you experience but how you interpret and respond to it that makes a difference. This means that your personal reaction to situations that are stressful can make an important difference in your health and well-being.

One might suggest that the easiest solution would be to avoid stressful situations as much as possible. This is what you try to do when you go on vacation, which is in itself filled with stress (packing, making arrangements etc.). The reality is that life itself is a struggle to maintain equilibrium. The deviations are what can excite, stimulate, and inspire you—but if you don't respond in a healthy, balanced way, stress will have a negative impact on your body.

As you might know, your life and environment are constantly changing, and for the majority of time, the circumstances and people you are involved with are beyond your power to change or control.

Since you can't change others, you need to concentrate on changing yourself. You can begin by changing the way you react to stressful situations. In many instances, it is your beliefs and attitudes that determine how you will respond to stressful situations. If that is the case, it might be time to consider reframing your point of view.

"Rigid beliefs, a tendency to prejudge (prejudice), and making or avoiding decisions because of shame, fear, or guilt create imbalance. Fear, shame, and guilt are distractions that cloak reality in a veil of illusion," said Dr. Nancy Iankowitz, Reiki practitioner, family nurse practitioner, and director of Holistic and Integrative Healing LLC. "*I have discovered that once people feel safe in an environment with a trusted mentor or guide, they are often able to let go of fear and see clearly. Then, through honest self-reflection, they may evaluate their responses to what they are suddenly aware of—separating truth from fiction, reality from illusion; these, once identified, help us heal as we reestablish the balance that the mind, body, and spirit strive to regain.*"

More than 50% of your stress in life comes from within you - not from outside. Your attitude and self-doubt are what prevent you from redefining yourself. Regretting past decisions and worrying about the future, prevent you from appreciating and enjoying your present.

Calm Your Mind to Relieve Stress

A great stress-relieving technique is to learn and practice the power of relaxation and to calm your mind. Meditation is one way of doing these things. According to Dr. Iankowitz, "*A deep, cleansing breath facilitates meditation, helping my patients balance their thoughts as they calm the mind. The first step would be to identify what one believes triggers the personal stress response. The next step is to reframe the personal reaction to it by putting it in perspective."*

An exercise I encourage you to do is to write down six major things in your life that you believe are a major cause of stress for you. Perhaps among these would be your job, a relationship, self-esteem issues or self-doubt. Maybe you have a pessimistic or overenthusiastic view of life or are easily disappointed by people around you.

Examine yourself to discover if you have rigid beliefs and attitudes that get in the way of peaceful living. Maybe you have annoying neighbors or in-laws. No matter how ridiculous your source of stress sounds, write it down. You can't fix the problem until you know what caused it. Once you complete your list, look it over, and next to each line, write down why or how the person or situation is stressful for you. Examine how you react every time you see that person or are faced with that situation, and write it down.

Then, once the list is completed and your reflective observations are noted, think about what you can do to reframe your response—unless, of course, it is actually possible to change the situation itself. Is it possible to change the situation? How serious is it? If your major stress is your work environment, what could be changed about your work or yourself to make it less stressful? Is changing your job an option?

There is a saying that if you can't do what you love; you will need to learn to love what you do. If changing your job is not an option for you right now, maybe instead of complaining all the time and being miserable, you could work on finding ways to change your attitude and your environment.

The Healing Power of Meditation

Meditation is often referred to as the art of being still; it is intended to purify your mind of thoughts that trigger your stress response—the reaction that keeps you in emotional and physical bondage. Meditation may help you achieve a state of self-awareness and tranquility, giving your body much needed rest and balance.

Meditation is an ancient practice dating as far back as 2,500 years; evidence-based research on the benefits of meditation confirms that this as a valuable and vital intervention. Recent published studies suggest that the benefits of meditation include relief from symptoms associated with conditions such as asthma, depression, heart disease, anxiety disorders, cancer, pain, high blood pressure, and sleep problems. Research also confirms there are different physiological changes occurring in the body during meditation, affecting systems such as the endocrine, metabolic, neurological and respiratory systems. Meditation has been shown to cause changes and slowing of brain waves, leading to calmness and balance.

There are many styles of meditation including the following:

Concentration meditation involves quieting and focusing your mind. It's the foundation of other forms of meditation.

Mindfulness meditation encourages you to focus on your thoughts and emotions as they move through your mind, assessing them without judgment.

Qi Gong and Tai Chi are forms of meditation with roots in Chinese medicine. They combine deep breathing with physical exercise to restore balance.

Transcendental meditation is a simple form of meditation where you repeat a personally assigned mantra—a word or a sound—to quiet your thoughts and achieve rest, relaxation, and inner peace.

Walking meditation is a form of meditation in action, using your movement of walking to turn your focus as you breathe with your footsteps.

Guided Meditation is led by a teacher who guides you to use your imagination to help calm and relax your thoughts and balance your mind.

Meditation is an activity that is easy to perform. It doesn't need equipment but does require time, space, and practice. You can try different types of meditation first to see which one best fits you and your lifestyle. You can sign up to attend classes with a group of people or practice meditation by yourself. In the beginning, you will probably benefit by guided meditation, where a teacher talks you through the correct technique. You can also use free websites such as www.learningmeditation.com_ and www.chopra.com_, both of which offer guided meditations. You can meditate for a few minutes at first, and then as you progress, increase the length of your meditation as needed. You can mediate at home, at work, or while walking in the park; all you need is a quiet place to concentrate. A simple meditation technique is outlined in 10 steps below:

- Find a quiet, safe place to meditate.
- Sit comfortably with your back straight and hands in your lap.
- Close your eyes, and (with your imagination) choose an object to concentrate on.
- Picture your chosen object (this may be a crystal or any symbol); focus on your breathing.
- Breathe slowly and deeply; breathe in for 4 counts, hold for 4, and out for 8.
- Let your feelings, emotions, and thoughts slowly drift in your mind.
- Keep your mind focused on the chosen object.

- Meditate for the amount of time you choose.
- Slowly bring your consciousness back to your surroundings.
- Open your eyes, and move slowly to get up.

Meditation is a form of exercise for your brain to help you to control your mind and your thoughts. Meditating regularly can help you to recover from the impact of a stressful lifestyle as it helps to improve your ability to cope with your life challenges. Start meditating regularly to find inner peace and calm your busy mind. I would like to finish this section with a quote from Mahatma Gandhi:

Keep your thoughts positive because your thoughts become your WORDS.
Keep your words positive because your words become your BEHAVIOR.
Keep your behavior positive because your behavior becomes your HABITS.
Keep your habits positive because your habits become your VALUES.
Keep your values positive because your values become your DESTINY.

Chapter 2

REDEFINING YOUR MIND — THE ART OF SELF-AWARENESS

"Your visions will become clear only when you can look into your own heart. Who looks outside, dreams; who looks inside, awakes." Carl Jung

Defining Self-Awareness

What is self-awareness? What is this magical word that promises happiness and tranquility? Does it exists, and can a busy woman have the time and a place for it in her life? Does it come from your mind or your heart? Self-awareness is defined and influenced by your inner core. It defines who you are, and it defines your perception of thoughts, beliefs, attitudes, and emotions. Self-awareness helps you to define who you want to be and what your purpose and goal in life is. Self-awareness is a powerful weapon that can be used to master and improve your mind, your thinking, and your life. You might ask where that self-awareness is hiding and why you've never met or seen it before.

Self-awareness is hiding deep inside you, waiting for you to tap into it and unlock its power. Every woman, busy or not, has that inner power, that inner feminine goddess living inside her. This busy woman's inner goddess is a cocoon with a beautiful butterfly inside waiting to unfurl its wings and fly. Your inner goddess could help you to become alive and free, loving and enjoying every moment of your life. Your inner goddess is sensual, feminine, and magnificent; it radiates positive thoughts, energy, and enthusiasm. It defines and knows your value and self-worth. It recognizes your flaws and your strengths. It could help you to spread your love to others and to receive love from others. Your inner goddess radiates warmth and beauty, passion and sexuality. Do you know your inner goddess; are you aware of her existence? If not, it is not too late. It is never too late to look deep inside yourself and unlock your inner goddess. It is not easy to define self-awareness; it could be terrifying to look inside yourself not knowing what you will find. Developing self-awareness takes time and practice until it becomes a habit and second nature to you.

Expanding Self-Awareness

To expand and develop your self-awareness you will need to learn to be present and to be consciously aware of your thoughts, feelings, emotions, and desires. You will need to slow down your thoughts and calm your feelings, trying to assess, analyze, and understand them. It is important to answer these questions while you are trying to understand yourself:

Where are these emotions and thoughts coming from? What and who are they influenced by? Do they represent who you are and what you believe in? What feelings are you experiencing with your thoughts? Do you experience anger and frustration or love and happiness? Why are you experiencing these particular emotions? What are these feelings influenced by?

As you can see, the list of questions is long and incomplete. Only you can know the answers to these questions. Deep breathing and meditation might be one way of calming your mind and gaining the opportunity to assess your thoughts and expand your self-awareness. When your mind is calm, you can look at your behavior and attitude and find out why are you having particular thoughts in certain situations and what your reaction to them is. Developing self-awareness will help you to change the thoughts in your mind, your interpretation of the situation, and the feelings you experience.

We all have positive and negative experiences in our lives, which often times consciously and unconsciously define and shape our behaviors and attitudes. Every reaction and feeling that we experience in any given situation is defined by our past experiences. This doesn't mean that we have to sit around and blame other people for our behavior. The Dalai Lama has an excellent quote: *"We can let the circumstances of our lives harden us so that we become increasingly resentful and afraid; or we can let them soften us, and make us kinder. We always have the choice."*

You would benefit greatly and improve your life if you identify your negative behavior, realize which feeling is causing it, and try to change your interpretation of the event and the feeling you are experiencing. For instance, listen to your self-talk. What are your thoughts and beliefs about yourself? Are they positive or negative? Who do you see in the mirror? Do you see the beautiful divine goddess that's who you are or somebody else with a list of imperfections and with self-doubt? Your negative thinking and self-doubt could get in the way of your accomplishments in life. Do you have a goal you wanted to reach or wished for something that you wanted to have for a long time but keep putting off trying to obtain them because you believe they are almost unattainable for you? Do you feel like this goal is behind a tall fence and you don't have what it takes to climb that fence? What you need to do is to assess and analyze what is causing your negative belief and self-doubt. What is stopping you from at least trying to reach that goal? Who and what are building this fence and making it higher and more difficult to climb? Is this fence actually as tall as you believe it to be, or are your fears and self-doubt making it impossible to climb it over? You could live the rest of your life in the shade of that fence. Or you could learn to look inside yourself, expand your self-awareness, conquer your fears and negative thoughts, and unlock your inner goddess with the wings of a butterfly. Who knows, you might be able to fly over that fence and reach your goal.

Living Your Life Purpose

Developing self-awareness and learning who you really are could help you obtain your purpose in life. Self-awareness can help you define your inner talents and gifts, which you can embrace to live fully in the moment and design the life you want. How do you know what your life purpose is? Look deep inside you, and your inner goddess will point you in the right direction. Living your life purpose means living happily. It means you are engaged in the activity that you love; you are surrounded by people that love you. It means enjoying every moment of your life. How do you find that elusive life purpose? How do you know it is the right one, and you were meant to live it?

You and only you can define what life purpose means to you and what you would like your life purpose to be. If you know your life purpose and are living it to the fullest, it is great and inspiring. I hope you are radiating happiness and sharing it with others. If you believe you don't know what your life purpose is yet, that is fine. You will find it eventually or might have already found it, and it is just taking you time to realize it. How do you find your life purpose? It might not be as complicated as you think. My grandmother had an excellent saying: *"You only have one life to live, and it is very short, so don't waste your time on things that are not meaningful to you."*

So to help you find your life purpose, I would like you to take some time and identify what is personally meaningful to you. Look inside yourself to see what your passions are. What are your values and beliefs? What strengths do you have? What are your weaknesses? Who is the person you want to or are trying to be? I would also like to ask you to look at your life now. I am sure as a busy woman, your life is like an overfilled cup, and you feel stretched beyond your human capacity. You are probably juggling being a mother, working, studying, taking care of the house and your family, and being present for a spouse, parents, and friends all at once. Probably the last thing on your mind right now is to start looking for your life purpose and adding more responsibilities to your busy life. But this situation might not necessarily be the case for you; you might be living your life purpose already and not realize it yet. I would like you to look at your life and see it differently, see it beyond the endless tasks and responsibilities, beyond the major and minor crises at school, work, or home.

I would like you to see where you personally are in this never-ending circuit of life. Where is that woman, that sensual, feminine, and magnificent goddess? Is she happy with the way her life is? Is this the type of life she dreamed about when she was younger? Happiness usually comes from living a life you believe you are meant to live. Ask yourself; are you truly happy with your life? Why not? Do you believe that if you are a stay-at-home mom, it is not what you were meant to be? Do you believe that working full time, going to school, and having a family at the same time was never on a list of your future life goals when you were a child?

If you don't have a career and are spending your life supporting your life partner, isn't that important? If you are busy going to college and taking care of your parents and loved ones, isn't it your life goal? Before you answer yes to these questions, please think about and write down what life purpose and fulfillment mean to you now and then when you will be 80 years old. Are they the same? Now write down what brings you joy in your life and how often you are able to have these things. Would this list change in 30–50 years?

As a mother, it can be difficult to keep perspective and not be angry when you are tired at night from cooking and cleaning, reading bedtime stories, helping with history homework and a chemistry lab report. But aside these difficulties, what could be more joyful than holding and hugging your child in your lap and read a story or play together? What is more precious than watching your children grow, succeed in school, and leave your house to go to college and to enter their own world? What do you think you will remember when you are 80 years old? Will you remember the tiredness and resentment of being a mother, or will you cherish the tender moments of love and kindness with your children? What do you think will give you a feeling of fulfillment? Would you think then that being a mother was not your life purpose? What I would like to suggest for you as a busy woman, mother, sister, daughter, and life partner is to open yourself to the present, and enjoy the privilege of sharing your life with others.

While you are taking care of you sick parents, instead of being angry and resentful, cherish these moments and save them in your memory. The time will come when your parents will not be with you anymore. If your college work and education is very stressful, focus on enjoying moments of quiet and peace while you are studying in the library; enjoy and cherish friendships and the knowledge that you are acquiring while being a student. While you give yourself selflessly to others and spread your love, I would also like you to remember that you are a woman with your own identity and your own sense and vision of purpose for your life.

My grandmother shared with me her own understanding of life purpose: *"Your life is your journey, which you take one step at a time. You should live your life in a way so when you look back, you have only good memories; when you look in the future, it is with purpose and excitement; when you look at present, it is with love and gratitude, and when you look inside yourself, it is for honesty and understanding."* So busy ladies, your life purpose is what you make of it. Let's live life to the fullest, enjoying every moment and collecting good memories for the future.

PART II

HEALING THE BODY

Chapter 3

BALANCING A WOMAN'S HORMONAL ORCHESTRA

"The more you worry the more you throw off the delicate balance of hormones required for health." Andrew Bernstein

Our hormones play a major role in our body functions and metabolism. They regulate multiple chemical reactions and help us to maintain homeostasis and internal balance. Our hormones have a unique way of communicating with each other. The Eastern medicine paradigm sees the body as a balance between forces of Yin and Yang. Western medicine holds that the body functions as a result of compensatory mechanisms and biofeedback. Our body's *temperature regulation* is one example of this. Did you ever think about why you perspire when you are outside in the hot weather? It happens because your body is trying to compensate. Perspiration is like a sprinkler system that cools the body. The body perspires through the skin as a way to cool down—decreasing your body temperature. This mechanism of "perspiring" also kicks in when we "break a fever." That is, after we run a fever, and the illness is successfully fought off, the body decides it doesn't need a high internal temperature anymore. A complex inner communication signals to the body that it is time to cool down. The body responds by setting off a "cool down sprinkler system" that we call "breaking a fever"—also referred to as "breaking out in a sweat." Similarly, when we shiver, that is also a compensatory mechanism. It happens when the body understands through its complex internal communication system that we have lost too much heat and need to warm up. The muscles rub together (the way we rub our hands together to warm up), and the result is "shivering" of the muscles involved. Cooling off and warming up are examples of how the body is able to compensate and balance temperature, and it happens automatically as a result of an appropriate, well-functioning internal feedback system. If the body is exposed to prolonged stress or trauma, eventually this compensatory mechanism is depleted, resulting in an imbalance.

In today's world, the hustle and bustle of daily life often creates a challenge for those of us with chaotic schedules. Specifically, we often find we are doing too much and not taking enough time to relax and nourish our body. An example would be that we are too rushed to eat a properly, well-balanced, nourishing meal. Am I right? Do you notice yourself doing this? Perhaps you grab something at a snack bar or have a piece of candy with a promise that a more substantial meal will follow (which may or may not happen). Today is a good day to plan to address this issue. Those of us with the talent and coordination to properly plan a meal and consume all the required daily nutrients might find it more difficult to nourish the soul. That is, even if you "eat right" you might be neglecting the deep breathing, stretching exercises, or other vital components needed to feed your soul. Do you take time to laugh each day? Do you find several minutes each day to take a mental vacation? If so—that is WONDERFUL! If not, pat yourself on the back for at least having read this far. This book is a positive, nourishing, and essential tool to feed your soul and your mind. Feeding the mind, body, and soul helps our hormones in their effort to work effectively in order to compensate and maintain the balance that the body requires to function optimally. Unfortunately, after prolonged exposure to stress (physical or emotional), hormones become imbalanced. The healthcare profession is seeing more and more people with chief complaints involving vague symptoms such as fatigue, insomnia, mood swings, anxiety, and unexplained body aches, to name a few. These reflect the imbalances we have been discussing so far.

Women are especially sensitive to these hormonal imbalances. In my practice, I have seen women who complain of hot flashes—even at the tender age of 30 (which is too early for menopause, in most cases). Women complain of painful, irregular periods, unexplained infertility, and a long list of other symptoms. Most of these women have one thing in common: they are very busy taking care of their career, family, children, and parents. In doing everything for everyone else, they often neglect themselves. In this chapter, I will discuss different hormonal imbalances that women most commonly experience.

Before I go into detail, let's review a few basics involving the female body's endocrine system. This is a complex communication network responsible for hormone secretion and regulation. I truly believe that in order to heal our imbalances, we need to first understand what is wrong. Then we could take action, which often involves learning about and understanding why it is important to follow a specific diet regimen or take a particular medication. The endocrine system is very complex; I will try to keep it very simple and straightforward so you have a basic understanding of how it works.

Meet The Master Glands: The Hypothalamus and Pituitary Gland

As mentioned above, the body is regulated by multiple biofeedback mechanisms that send messengers such as hormones through a network of internal pathways. The hormones travel throughout the body in order to regulate its functions and help the body adjust to change. The body produces approximately 100 different hormones that communicate with and depend on each other. If one hormone becomes imbalanced, very often, the impact is felt by other hormones in the communication network, resulting in a compensatory mechanism that either over- or under-produces related hormones. As in a domino effect, many hormones eventually react, causing a hormonal cascade of connected symptoms and problems.

The **hypothalamus** is the body's master gland. It is responsible for coordinating all the hormones, including the growth hormone (GH), oxytocin, and prolactin. These are among the many hormones that serve as messengers, and they are all constantly interacting. The hypothalamus gives direct orders to its sister gland—the *pituitary gland*, which in turn regulates other glands in the body such as the *adrenal gland, thyroid gland*, the *ovaries* in women, and *testes* in men. The connection between the hypothalamus, pituitary, and other glands is called a *hypothalamic-pituitary-endocrine axis* (HPEA). The pathway between the hypothalamus and the pituitary-adrenal gland is called an HPA axis.

The **pituitary gland** is a small pea-shaped organ located at the base of the brain behind the bridge of the nose/center of the forehead. It is responsible for sensing changes in the body and sending signals to other glands, telling them to regulate their function in order to reestablish or maintain a balanced environment. For example, the pituitary gland produces the thyroid-stimulating hormone (TSH), which acts on the thyroid gland to induce the production of the thyroid hormones T_3 and T_4. The pituitary gland also secretes hormones that regulate the adrenal gland, testes, and ovaries, which in turn produce other hormones.

For the purposes of this book, I will focus on three major glands that affect woman's health extensively: the thyroid, adrenal, and ovaries. There is a very close and sometimes opposing relationship between these glands and the hormones they secrete. This relationship is called an Ovarian Adrenal Thyroid (OAT) axis. When one group of hormones—let's say the stress hormones—is out of balance, it causes imbalances with sex hormones and thyroid hormones. For example, if a woman has her ovaries removed, both the adrenal and thyroid gland functions are affected. The female body needs all three glands to be balanced and functioning properly in order to be in optimal health and to feel great. Dr. Hyla Cass and Kathleen Barnes published an excellent book on female hormonal imbalances entitled *8 Weeks to Vibrant Health.* In her book, Dr. Cass offers a wealth of information on different hormonal imbalances that women experience and their effects on the body in various topics including brain chemistry, premenstrual syndrome (PMS), menopause, imbalances of thyroid and adrenal glands, metabolic syndrome, blood sugar imbalances, and much more. She also provides readers with detailed natural treatment protocols to help correct imbalances, reclaim energy, and restore well-being.   Before I make it more complicated, let's take a look at each of these glands in a bit more detail.

THE SUPER HEROES — ADRENAL GLANDS

Adrenal glands are two triangular shaped glands located on the kidneys that consist of an outer cortex and an inner medulla. They are fairly small in size but very powerful and important in their tasks. They produce about 50 different hormones that are essential to optimum health. The adrenal glands are responsible for producing hormones that affect 4 major things in your body—Salt, Sugar, Stress, and Sex.

- Salt—aldosterone production regulates your water and electrolytes
- Sugar—cortisol production regulates the glucose metabolism in your body
- Stress—adrenalin production regulates your stress response
- Sex—DHEA and various sex hormone production regulates sex hormone precursors and characteristics

Two major hormones produced by the adrenal glands are cortisol and adrenalin. They work hand in hand and are continuously secreted to help regulate different physiological functions. Adrenalin is a short-acting hormone, released in a time of stress or emergency. Cortisol is a long-acting hormone, released after adrenalin, which lasts longer to support the body after the stress response is over. In order to understand the importance of adrenal glands and their hormonal response during stress, let's first understand what stress is and how it affects the body.

What Is Stress?

We busy women are all too familiar with stress as it is a constant companion in our busy schedules. Stress can be physical or emotional. It may be positive (facilitating) or negative (debilitating), depending on how we interpret it and react to it. In any situation, however, the stress response (release of stress hormones) causes the body to react, and unless we learn how to take conscious control, this reaction disturbs the body's normal physiological equilibrium.

So what happens in the body when we are under stress? I am sure each of us, at some point in our life, has been faced with an emergency situation in which we had to act quickly. During that situation, we were able to do something that we wouldn't have been able to do under normal circumstances; for example, jump over a high fence or run fast. Dr. Nancy Iankowitz, Director of Holistic and Integrative Healing LLC, recalls a time wherein she was 5 months pregnant with her second child when her 29-month-old daughter was suddenly on the other side of a 4-foot fence in their not-so-safe neighborhood in Queens, New York. Her stress response facilitated an automatic physical response. During our interview, she shared, "I scaled that fence, much to my own shock, as if I was light as a feather. All turned out well in that scenario; however, we need to help our patients be aware that the stress response is quite a powerful one."

What happened in the above scenario? The "fight-flight" response kicked in. This term was first described by Walter Cannon, a Harvard physiologist who explained it as our body's automatic, primitive, and inborn response to stress. It prepares our body to either face the threat and "fight" or flee by taking "flight" from a perceived attack. This response protected our cave-dwelling ancestors from the all too real saber-toothed tigers.

When faced with a perceived danger, a very complicated response triggers the release of a hormonal cascade that impacts multiple organs in the body. Hormones like adrenalin, noradrenalin, and cortisol are secreted. Our pupils dilate to improve our eyesight. Our lungs and the respiratory tree become dilated as well to improve the oxygen supply to our body. Our heart rate increases to improve blood circulation to our internal organs and muscles. At the same time, a big portion of our circulating blood is rerouted from our peripheral vasculature (arms and legs), digestive, and urinary tract and directed to our main internal organs (the brain, lungs, heart, liver, and kidneys). More blood and oxygen is supplied to our muscles in preparation for running (fleeing) as they require extra fuel and energy. Cortisol, released by the adrenal gland, stimulates the liver to convert saved glucagon into glucose so it may be utilized for energy. Our immune system becomes activated as well to help protect us if needed. The skin becomes cold, which decreases its chances of bleeding if it becomes cut during the fight or flight response. All these changes sharpen our sight, increase our awareness, and improve our reflexes and impulses. Our body is physically and psychologically prepared to react quickly in order to protect itself from the perceived enemy. This mechanism works well and helps us to survive in emergency situations.

The reality is that even if we don't live in a cave or have to fight off saber-toothed tigers, we do occasionally have a need for the fight-flight response. Dr. Iankowitz, mentioned earlier, jumped a 4-foot fence while 5-months pregnant when faced with what she perceived to be a crisis. We all hear unbelievable stories such as these on the news about fathers rescuing their children from fire or an accident. What is important to realize, though, is that the body reacts the same way to any small stress as well—even from something simple such as being stuck in traffic, being afraid of being late for work, or having a negative comment directed at us. Anything in our life (whether it is physical, psychological, or emotional) that we perceive as a threat has the potential to trigger that emergency response. In any perceived emergency, the body works extensively to protect us. Once the perceived threat is over, our body regulates the stress hormone production to reestablish balance and internal calm. Ideally, as the body returns to a state of calm, the heart rate returns to normal, blood pressure decreases, and our muscles relax—all in response to decreased anxiety as our mind becomes calm once again.

Unfortunately, our hectic modern life presents us with a series of small, constantly stressful situations. As noted above, our body reacts to each situation the same way; it doesn't know the difference between "life threatening emergency situations" and "mild daily stress." Our adrenals are constantly working. If they don't get a chance to rest, they eventually become imbalanced. Adrenal glands may become exhausted and unable to function properly, releasing suboptimal amounts of hormones. This may potentially lead to disorders involving a hormonal imbalance or immune system dysfunction as is often seen in depression, which is expressed as an increased susceptibility to infections. Adrenal exhaustion can also cause chronic fatigue, allergies, and autoimmune disorders such as lupus and multiple sclerosis.

Adrenal glands may also become overactive and release hormones at inappropriate times, causing myriad symptoms including headaches, heart palpitations, anxiety, insomnia, high blood pressure, and irritable bowel syndrome. Adrenal fatigue may also result from physiological conditions such as chronic illness or pain, sleep deprivation, chronic or acute infection, high sugar intake, strenuous exercise, undetected food sensitivities and depression. Constant stress placed upon the body drains our adrenal glands, and this problem coupled with a stressful lifestyle predisposes a person to adrenal fatigue and exhaustion. At this point, I think it's time to define *adrenal fatigue*, explain how it presents itself, and review the symptoms of this condition as well as how it is diagnosed and treated.

Adrenal Fatigue

Adrenal fatigue doesn't occur overnight. It usually happens gradually as a response to chronic exposure to physiological stressors. Examples of this would be an overfilled schedule precluding the adequate intake of nutrients, a lifestyle that deprives us of enough sleep, and overexposure to emotional stressors, including our failure to take a few minutes for ourselves to meditate, stretch, and breathe deeply. These factors combine to slowly drain our adrenal glands, resulting in the imbalanced production of hormones.

Unfortunately, imbalanced adrenal hormones also have a significant effect on other glands in the body and affect their hormonal production as well. For instance, abnormal levels of *cortisol* directly affect insulin levels, blood glucose regulation, and the production of hormones such as *ghrelin* and *leptin*, which are responsible for our feelings of hunger and fullness. As a result of these imbalances, we experience food cravings and weight gain. Constant exposure to stress also affects our sex hormones and leads to symptoms such as painful periods, PMS, and decreased libido. Hormones secreted by the adrenals also have a great impact on thyroid gland hormones, causing imbalances in metabolism and symptoms such as weight gain, decreased energy, and changes in mood.

Three Stages of Adrenal Imbalance

The first stage is characterized by the overproduction of cortisol triggered by a lot of stress, as when one is juggling several responsibilities and, though feeling fatigued, is unable to rest and relax. If you are in this situation, you might experience poor sleep, anxiety, agitation, or may also suffer from gastrointestinal issues such as bloating, constipation, nausea, indigestion, and reflux. Perhaps you have a weak immune system. Over time, for those who neglect self-care or otherwise fail to alleviate or at least control the perception of daily stress, the adrenals eventually get tired, setting the body up for the second stage of adrenal fatigue.

The second stage is characterized by a decline in cortisol production. The tired adrenals are unable to produce a sufficient amount of cortisol throughout the day. In this stage, one characteristically exhibits symptoms of general fatigue. Those who turn to stimulants such as caffeine to help keep them going might experience some unexplained bodily aches and pains. This is the body saying, "I resent being neglected." Caffeine addresses a symptom: fatigue. But the root cause is an adrenal problem as in a hormonal imbalance. Avoiding the root cause sets us up for continued issues. Your body might get tired easily, lack energy even after a full night's sleep, or may be prone to infection, which further drains the adrenal glands. You might begin to gain unexplained weight and experience problems with your sex drive, which will decline over time.

During **the third stage**, the adrenal glands produce a very small amount of hormones that barely peak during the day. The person feels extremely weak, has no energy, and can't even perform simple daily activities. Individuals in stage three often rely heavily on stimulants to get through the day.

Your Adrenal Reserves

Your adrenals are affected by a wide variety of physical, mental, and emotional factors. The table below lists things that will drain your adrenal reserves, and things that you could do to support and rejuvenate your adrenals.

Drain adrenals	Rejuvenate adrenals
Physical drains:	*Physical support:*
Not enough or poor quality of sleep	Sleep at least 7–8 hours/night
Fasting: missed meals	Breathing exercises
Caffeine and all stimulants	Meditation
Alcohol	Tai Chi, Yoga
Smoking	Quit smoking and drinking alcohol
Food allergies	Massage
Infections	Reiki, body work, Rolfing
Refined sugars	Eat nourishing foods every 2–3 hours
Food additives and artificial sweeteners	Drink sufficient amounts of fluids
Toxins, heavy metals, pesticides, herbicides	Mild stretching and exercises
Prolonged and excessive exercises	Relaxation bath

Mental and Emotional drains	Mental and Emotional support
Feelings of anger or resentment	Positive self-talk
Worry	Releasing negative thoughts
Guilt	Feelings of Love and Joy
Grief	Peace
Fear	Courage
Shame	Life purpose
Unresolved conflict	Living in alignment of core beliefs;
Negative thoughts	Resolving relationship issues

Please use the left column of the chart below to list your physical, emotional, and mental stressors. In the right hand column, list things that may relieve some of the stressors you have in your life. Ask yourself these questions: What is draining my adrenals and my energy? Is it my lifestyle, relationships, or my work? Do I take time to enjoy myself and enjoy life? What could I do to relieve stress and improve and restore my adrenal reserves?

Stress producing	Stress relieving

Can Adrenal Fatigue Be Healed?

If you suspect you may be suffering from adrenal fatigue, don't panic. The good news is that there are multiple treatments available. First, you need to find a health care practitioner who is trained to treat adrenal fatigue. Your practitioner will take a detailed medical history, ask questions about your diet and lifestyle, and will then order some diagnostic tests. Your practitioner will probably ask you to fill out a food diary to obtain detailed information about your eating habits. Your practitioner might order the following tests:

- Saliva test to measure levels of cortisol, DHEA, and other hormones
- Blood test to measure levels of thyroid hormones such as TSH, free T_3 and T_4, total and reverse T_3, and thyroid antibodies
- Fasting insulin and sugar levels with a 3–4 hour glucose tolerance test
- Other blood tests to measure your blood count, electrolytes, cholesterol levels, vitamin levels, and much more

Dr. Cass offers a self-test, easily performed at home, to assess adrenal fatigue. According to Dr. Cass, "You would need a blood pressure cuff or monitor and a helper. Lie on your back for at least 5 minutes. Then have your helper record your blood pressure. Sit up quickly, and have your blood pressure recorded again. Then stand up quickly and take it again. In people without adrenal dysfunction, blood pressure will rise between 4 to 10 points with each measurement. If your blood pressure drops, it is likely that you have adrenal exhaustion."

While you wait for your appointment and test results, there is a lot you can do on your own. Since adrenal fatigue doesn't occur overnight, it is not "fixed" overnight either. It will take time and effort on your part to repair and heal yourself. Please be patient. This book offers many tools to help you recover so you can feel great again.

What Can I Do To Heal My Adrenals?

Since busy women have lives so full of activities and responsibilities, it is almost impossible for us to avoid all stressful situations. To protect our adrenals, it is important to learn how to deal effectively with stressful situations. There are several things you can start doing today to relieve some of your stress.

First, it is important to nourish your body. Begin by eating high quality nourishing meals throughout the day. Try to eat fresh whole foods that are organic, including lots of fruits and vegetables. Never skip breakfast; rather, within an hour of rising, try to eat a breakfast that includes a source of protein. This habit replenishes glucose stores that were depleted during the night—an important beginning for an energetic day.

Time your meals so that you have a healthy "small meal" or snack every 2-3 hours. This helps avoid low blood sugar and prevents the energy crash that contributes to food cravings. (read more about food cravings in Chapter 5). Avoid drinking beverages that contain caffeine and alcohol, as they drain the adrenals and actually exacerbate symptoms. (Avoid so called energy drinks such as Red Bull since they are very destructive to the internal balance you are trying to restore). Herbal caffeine-free teas such as chamomile, passionflower and valerian are very calming and support your adrenals. The following chapters of this book provide you with detailed information on types of diets available and the importance of following a well-balanced diet. Part 4 of this book provides you with healthy, easy to make recipes you might include in your diet.

Another important factor in healing adrenal fatigue is adequate, quality sleep. Sleep helps restore the body, improves metabolism and rejuvenates adrenals. Chapter 7 of this book discusses the importance of adequate sleep, and provides you with information and tools to improve your sleeping habits.

Getting sufficient exercise might also help relieve stress, which is a key factor in healing your adrenals. Exercise might help to balance your cortisol levels and decrease insulin resistance. The exercise chapter of this book offers a wealth of information on types of exercise regimens available and offers tips on how to appropriately choose an exercise program that best suits your health and lifestyle. Depending on your stage of adrenal fatigue, your exercise regimen might need to be adjusted. Those experiencing stage 2 or 3 should avoid vigorous aerobic exercise. Vigorous exercises put more stress on your tired adrenals and can make the condition worse. If you don't feel energized after your exercise routine, chances are these exercise are not right for you. The recommendation is that you consider more gentle walking exercises while receiving treatment to support your adrenals, and increase your activity as your condition improves.

Balancing your emotional and mental stress will speed the healing process for your adrenals. Dr. Iankowitz shared this tip during our interview: "I help my patients to reframe stressors so that the perception of whatever they are facing or having to deal with can be put into proper perspective. For example, if a person breaks a fingernail, unless that person is a hand model, this event should not cause a tremendous stress response. (If that person happens to be a hand model, then taking a deep breath goes a long way since oxygen in the blood signals to the brain that we can handle the stressor and don't need a rush of cortisol.")

Try to set aside some time during the day for yourself. It is important to spend at least 10–15 minutes of quiet time—a perfect opportunity to center yourself. Meditation is one of the ways to find the balance necessary to heal. Letting go of past hurts, avoiding villain/victim/savior scenarios, forgiving yourself and others for disappointments you have experienced/shared, and resolving past relationship issues that might be a constant, nagging weight or burden on your mind might help you to get rid of unnecessary emotional stressors.

Another effective intervention to help restore your adrenals is to eliminate the environmental toxins and chemicals that bombard your body on a daily basis. These are pesticides, herbicides, synthetic colors and pigments, artificial food coloring and flavors, artificial sweeteners, parabens, heavy metals, petrochemicals, hydrogenated oils, HFCS (high fructose corn syrup), and many, many more. In Part 4 of this book, you are provided with detailed information on environmental toxins and the best ways to clean your environment. After considering all aforementioned interventions, your health care practitioner might prescribe a treatment consisting of herbal supplements, nutritional vitamins and minerals, and bioidentical hormones. Dr. Cass recommends commonly used herbal supplements to support adrenals such as Ashwagandha, Eleuthero/ Siberian Ginseng, Phosphorylated Serine or Phosphatidylserine, Reishi mushroom, and Licorice root.

Other supplements used to support adrenals are vitamin C and vitamin B complex. Please don't attempt to treat yourself at home with these supplements. Their dosages vary greatly based on the stage of adrenal fatigue you have and your individual medical conditions. A well-trained health care provider will prescribe an appropriate regimen based on your diagnostic results and your symptoms. Adrenal recovery might take you anywhere from 6 months to 2 years. Please be patient and persistent; adapt slowly to the changes we discuss in this book, and soon you would feel much better, with renewed energy to enjoy your life.

THYROID GLAND — YOUR ENERGY MACHINE

The thyroid gland is located in the front of the neck, and it has two sides or lobes. This tiny butterfly-shaped organ is a powerful energy and metabolism machine in our body. It affects almost all body functions and regulates the metabolism, which turns food into energy. If the thyroid gland is malfunctioning and not producing enough hormones, our whole body slows down causing symptoms such as lethargy, fatigue, constipation, and intolerance to cold. An overactive thyroid, on the other hand, can cause symptoms of an increased metabolism such as anxiety, agitation, heart palpitations, and intolerance to heat. Let's take a look at how the thyroid gland functions.

The thyroid gland is influenced by the hypothalamus and pituitary glands, which together create the hypothalamic-pituitary-thyroid axis. The hypothalamus produces a thyrotropin releasing hormone (TRH), which stimulates the pituitary gland to produce the thyroid stimulating hormone (TSH). TSH then stimulates the thyroid gland to release hormones thyroxine (T4) and triiodothyronine (T3).

These hormones are essential for life and have numerous effects on body growth, metabolism, and development. Our body self-regulates the production of TSH, TRH, T3, and T4 with a biofeedback mechanism. For instance, if levels of thyroid hormones T3 and T4 drop in the bloodstream, the hypothalamus detects it and releases TRH, stimulating the pituitary gland to produce TSH. Rising levels of TSH will stimulate the thyroid gland to produce more T3 and T4, eventually returning the thyroid hormone levels in the blood back to normal. The thyroid gland acts like the body's sensory barometer. The main function of the thyroid is converting calories and oxygen into energy. It helps to regulate blood pressure, metabolism, body temperature, growth, and heart rate.

The American Thyroid Association (ATA) states that thyroid disorders are on the rise, and an estimated 20 million Americans have some form of thyroid disease. More than 12% of people in the US develop a thyroid condition during their lifetime. Up to 60% of those with thyroid disease are unaware of their condition. Women are 5–8 times more likely than men to have thyroid problems.

Dr. Dana Cohen, an Integrative Medicine Physician, says she treats a wide variety of patients in her practice for thyroid related health problems. Many of her patients have subclinical hypothyroidism, a condition where a person might exhibit all the symptoms but have normal blood levels. Dr. Cohen recommends that all women who might experience symptoms of abnormal thyroid function be tested routinely. Chronically undiagnosed thyroid disease may put patients at risk for certain serious conditions, such as cardiovascular diseases, osteoporosis, and infertility. The good news is most thyroid diseases can be successfully managed with appropriate medical attention.

Causes of Thyroid Dysfunction

There are multiple causes for thyroid dysfunction, starting with genetics. If you have a family member with a history of thyroid disease, your chances of developing a similar disease in the future are much higher. Other causes might include previous surgery to the thyroid gland and certain medications such as sulfa drugs, estrogen, birth control pills, lithium, and amiodarone.

The function of the thyroid gland is influenced greatly by iodine, which is the chief component of thyroid hormones and is important for their production. We obtain iodine from our diet, from the food we consume and the water we drink. It is very important to have a sufficient amount of iodine in our diet. Insufficient iodine intake can cause a decreased production of thyroid hormone and cause an enlargement of the thyroid gland, a condition called a goiter. On the other hand, taking excess amounts of iodine in foods such as kelp might aggravate autoimmune thyroid disease. Our toxic environment has a direct impact on our thyroid health. Excessive amounts of fluoride, chloride, and bromide added to our water and our food interfere with our iodine function, which might predispose us to decreased thyroid function.

There are more cases of hypothyroidism today and many researchers believe it may be directly related to the stressful lifestyles we live. There is a connection between the thyroid and adrenal gland that might explain why increased stress might affect your thyroid function. When you have low levels of thyroid hormones, your adrenal glands produce less cortisol in response. Cortisol is necessary for the production of T3 and T4. Your adrenal glands and thyroid glands influence each other, so if you have adrenal fatigue as discussed in the previous chapter, you might also develop a thyroid dysfunction. On the other hand, if you happen to have hypothyroidism, constant levels of low thyroid hormones will burden your adrenals and might cause adrenal fatigue.

Symptoms of Thyroid Dysfunction

Symptoms of thyroid dysfunction vary depending on an individual, and since adrenal fatigue often accompanies thyroid dysfunction, many of the symptoms of these two conditions overlap. Below is a partial list of the most common symptoms women with imbalanced thyroid hormones experience. You don't have to experience all of these symptoms to be diagnosed with a thyroid imbalance. Having only 3–4 symptoms might be a sufficient indication of your thyroid dysfunction.

Underactive Thyroid	Overactive Thyroid
Cold intolerance—especially hands and feet	Feeling hot
Constipation	Sweating
Weight gain	Problems falling asleep
Fatigue	Racing thoughts
Forgetfulness	Difficulty focusing
Decreased libido or sex drive	Forgetfulness
Dry hair and dry skin	Elevated heart rate and heart palpitations
Brittle nails	Anxiety, nervousness, or irritability
Muscle cramps	Fatigue
Depression	Weight loss
Decreased menstrual flow	Menstrual problems
Swelling in the front of the neck (goiter)	Change in bowel function—loose stool

Can A Thyroid Imbalance Be Healed?

If you suspect that you might be developing a thyroid imbalance, you are one step closer to your recovery. You can also perform a self-test at home to confirm your suspicions. To do this, you need a thermometer to perform a basal body temperature test. Check you temperature using a regular mercury thermometer early in the morning before you get out of bed. Hold the thermometer for 10 *minutes in* your armpit, and record your temperature. Repeat this test for at least 3 days. Make sure to perform this test when you are not ovulating, starting on day 3 of your cycle. Healthy individuals usually have a basal body temperature of 98.4° F and above. If your basal body temperature is below 97.8° F, you might have an underactive thyroid.

Next, find a health care practitioner in your area trained to treat a thyroid imbalance. Your health care practitioner will perform a detailed health history and physical assessment and order some diagnostic tests. Your practitioner might order the following tests:

A blood test to measure levels of thyroid hormones such as TSH, free T3 and T4, total and reverse T3, thyroid peroxidase antibodies, and antithyroid antibodies can be done. If you happen to have an enlarged thyroid gland, your provider might recommend an ultrasound of your thyroid to detect any cysts and nodules that you might have developed. A 24-hour urine collection might be ordered to check your iodine levels if your practitioner suspects you of having an iodine deficiency.

As discussed previously, thyroid and adrenal dysfunction affect each other most of the time. So it is very important to also check your adrenal function when your thyroid work up is being performed. While you are waiting for your appointment and test results, there is a lot you could do on your own to help you to heal your thyroid.

What Could I Do To Heal My Thyroid?

First, it is important to modify your diet and lifestyle to decrease your stress levels and to provide your body with enough support to heal itself, as was discussed in the previous chapter on adrenal fatigue. Aside from the general diet modifications recommended in this book, some foods affect thyroid gland function and should be restricted from your diet. Cruciferous vegetables such as broccoli, cauliflower, cabbage, mustard, and kale are considered goitrogenic, which means they might interfere with thyroid hormone production. Other products on the list are soy isoflavones, millet, strawberries, spinach, and peaches.

This is not a reason to panic and eliminate all above-mentioned products from your diet. To decrease the goitrogenic effects of cruciferous vegetables, you should eat them cooked or steamed; soy products should be fermented or cultured and paired with iodine containing seaweed products such as Kombu or Nori. Use your common sense, and eat a smaller portion of these products if you still have concerns.

Another effective way to restore your thyroid is to eliminate or decrease your exposure to products that have high levels environmental toxins such as fluoride, chloride, and bromide. Since these elements are present in tap water, purchasing a water filter is a good solution.

And finally, if the above-mentioned methods are not enough to restore your thyroid, your health care practitioner might prescribe you a treatment consisting of herbal supplements, nutritional vitamins and minerals, and bioidentical hormones.

Dr. Cohen uses an individual approach to help restore the thyroid function of her patients. She utilizes natural thyroid hormones, such as Nature-Throid among the others, to adjust the doses of the medication and achieve optimum results for the patient. Dr. Cohen also recommends testing and treating underlying adrenal fatigue while treating thyroid dysfunction. Thyroid medication causes an increase in metabolism and places an increased demand on adrenal function and cortisol production. Therefore, individuals with adrenal fatigue will not be able to meet the increased metabolic demand and will feel much worse after taking their thyroid medication. If this is the case, adrenal function should be restored first before initiating treatment for thyroid imbalance.

Other supplements that might benefit you if you have a thyroid imbalance include vitamins A, C, E, and B complex along with magnesium, selenium, iodine, zinc, and coenzyme Q_{10}. Ashwagandha is an adaptogenic herb that has been shown to benefit adrenal and thyroid gland function and is recommended to patients with those imbalances.

Please don't attempt to treat yourself at home with these supplements; their recommended dosages can vary greatly and must be based on your individual medical conditions. A trained health care provider will prescribe you an appropriate regimen based on your diagnostic results and your symptoms. Thyroid recovery might require a careful titration of your medication and monitoring of your symptoms. Please be patient and persistent; you now have all the information and tools needed to understand the connection between your adrenal and thyroid health. Contact your health care provider to start your treatment, and feel free to use information provided in this book to help you modify your lifestyle and your health.

OVARIES — MESSENGERS FROM VENUS

In previous chapters, we discussed the effect of stress and thyroid hormones on your body and on overall hormonal balance. In this chapter, I would like to discuss ovaries and sex hormones, which have a great influence on your well-being and functioning.

Ovaries

Each woman has two ovaries, which are part of her reproductive and endocrine systems. Ovaries have two main functions; the first is to produce ova for fertilization, and the second is to produce hormones such as estrogen and progesterone. The production of estrogen and progesterone in the ovaries is regulated by the hypothalamus, which releases gonadotropin-releasing hormone (GnRH). GnRH regulates the release of luteinizing hormone (LH) and follicle-stimulating hormone (FSH) from the pituitary gland. LH and FSH promote ovulation and regulate estrogen and progesterone secretion through the cycle.

Estrogen production dominates in the first half of your menstrual cycle—before ovulation—and progesterone production dominates during the second half of the menstrual cycle— when the corpus luteum has formed. Both hormones are important in the preparation of the lining of the womb (uterus) for pregnancy and the implantation of a fertilized egg (zygote), which after about two weeks becomes an embryo. Estrogen is responsible for your female characteristics, providing you with soft skin, a high-pitched voice, full breasts, and wide hips. Estrogen is produced by the ovaries, the adrenal glands, and in fat cells.

Progesterone is responsible for regulating your menstrual cycle, is important in maintaining a healthy pregnancy, and counterbalances the effects of estrogen in the body. Progesterone acts as the antagonist of estrogen. In Eastern medicine, estrogen and progesterone are considered the opposing forces of Yin (estrogen) and Yang (progesterone). They counterbalance and regulate each other through the monthly cycle of the female body. For example, estrogen might be responsible for the production of breast cysts while progesterone protects against breast cysts. Progesterone is considered a natural diuretic, while estrogen promotes water and salt retention.

This particular balance of these two hormones plays a big role in women's well-being. Problems arise, usually, when there is an imbalance between these two, when there is a dominance of one of these hormones. This imbalance is responsible for causing multiple symptoms that you might experience throughout your cycle. Let's see what happens during the menstrual cycle since this cycle is a great indicator of your hormonal balance:

The menstrual cycle is divided into 3 phases: estrogen phase, progesterone phase, and menstrual phase.

Estrogen phase. This phase begins during the week following your menstrual period when levels of estrogen begin to rise. It lasts 7–12 days and usually ends in ovulation. During this phase, you generally feel and look your best—no bloating, food cravings, or imbalanced moods. (These unpleasant experiences usually occur during the progesterone phase.) During the estrogen phase, your body prepares itself for ovulation and fertilization; nature helps you to focus on finding your mate and reproduce. This explains why a lot of women experience increased libido and sexual drive during this time of the month. Estrogen is also responsible, during this phase, for creating a clearer skin complexion and glossier hair. Your body metabolism is increased during this time; you might feel energized, attractive, and self-confident.

Progesterone phase. This phase begins during ovulation (days 14–16 of your menstrual cycle) and lasts about 2 weeks. During this phase, your body prepares for possible pregnancy. Your metabolism slows down, and your body becomes calm. Once the body realizes that there is no pregnancy, progesterone levels drop. This is the time when the majority of premenstrual symptoms develop.

Approximately 3–5 days before your "period" (the actual time of bleeding—shedding the accumulated lining preparation in the womb for pregnancy), your body goes into progesterone withdrawal, causing myriad symptoms including, irritability, anxiety, crying more easily, bloating, breast tenderness, swelling, and water retention. During this time, it is important to take care of yourself by using stress relieving techniques such as meditation to decrease agitation and to prevent confrontation. Use recommendations provided in Chapter 5 to avoid food cravings and to choose the most optimally nutritious foods that your body needs during this phase.

Menstrual phase. This phase begins the day you start bleeding and lasts 3–6 days while your uterus sheds its lining. During this phase, your levels of progesterone and estrogen hormones are relatively low; a hormone-like substance called prostaglandin is released at this time. As a result, your uterus experiences mild contractions to force the release of the lining it prepared in case you became pregnant. Your emotions become more stable during this time, while your body might experience discomfort such as cramping, headaches, and body aches.

You should honor your body and take some time to rest, if possible, during this period. The body needs extra support and nourishment at this special time. Most women experience mild, tolerable symptoms and minor discomfort through the three phases of the menstrual cycle; however, if your symptoms range from moderate to severe, this might be an indication that your hormones are out of balance.

Hormonal Imbalances

PMS — Premenstrual Syndrome. We have all heard of Premenstrual Syndrome (PMS), to which our not-so-pleasant days (including mood swings) are sometimes attributed. I often hear, "PMS doesn't exist," and claims that it is all in our head. Well, is it true? Is it all in our head? In helping you decide, I would like to share some information on PMS discovered during my research.

Premenstrual Syndrome – PMS is a condition involving a variety of symptoms (emotional, physical and behavioral) that are directly related to a woman's menstrual cycle and develop 7–10 days prior to your period. It is considered the luteal phase of the menstrual cycle during which time, as discussed above, there is shift of hormones from estrogen to progesterone. Some of the PMS symptoms might result from an interaction between progesterone and a brain neurotransmitters called serotonin (which is responsible for our mood stability).

Research shows that serotonin levels are much lower during the luteal phase in women with PMS. This fact might explain the symptoms of anxiety, moodiness, irritability, and depression that occur with this condition. Other symptoms of PMS, such as fluid retention and bloating, may be caused by the impact of progesterone and estrogen on kidney function, affecting the balance of salt and fluid retention in the body. Mild symptoms and discomfort experienced before and during the days you menstruate, even though unpleasant, might be a normal occurrence, says Daniel Roshan, MD, FACOG, FACS, Diplomat, American Board of OB/GYN/Maternal-Fetal Medicine and Director of Rosh Maternal Fetal Medicine in New York.

However, if you experience severe menstrual pain and heavy bleeding with clots, it warrants an evaluation by your gynecologist as these might be symptoms of more serious conditions such as endometriosis, uterine fibroids, or pelvic inflammatory disease. In addition, if behavioral and emotional symptoms are intense and interfere with daily activities, they might represent a more serious condition called premenstrual dysphoric disorder (PMDD). Dr. Roshan recommends that you see your health care provider if you have symptoms of hopelessness, despair, lack energy to perform your daily activities, and feel overwhelmed or out of control. PMDD is a more serious condition than PMS and warrants a careful diagnosis, medical treatment, and monitoring of symptoms.

Symptoms of PMS in cycling women usually develop 7–14 days before menstruation during the progesterone phase and might be linked to an insufficient production of progesterone. One of the most common contributing factors to low progesterone levels is stress. As discussed previously, our adrenal glands are responsible for our stress response by producing cortisol. The problem arises because adrenal glands require progesterone to produce cortisol. If you are constantly under a high degree of stress, and your adrenal glands are required to produce high levels of cortisol, they do it by robbing your body of progesterone. Thus, the progesterone produced by your ovaries is not enough to regulate your reproductive functions. This deficiency of progesterone makes the situation worse by causing an imbalance involving estrogen, progesterone, and testosterone. This imbalance may represent another condition called estrogen dominance—a topic discussed in greater detail later on in this chapter.

On the other hand, when cortisol levels are constantly elevated, they cause a decrease in the production of progesterone in the ovaries as well as interrupt progesterone activity by competing for the same receptor sites to enter the cells. As we can see, stress disrupts our hormonal balance and causes PMS, and PMS symptoms themselves put a lot of stress on our body and affect our adrenal glands. This process becomes a vicious cycle and needs to be addressed—the sooner the better.

What Can I Do About PMS?

Mild symptoms of PMS may be successfully relieved by simple changes in your lifestyle and some home remedies. To relieve pain and cramping during your period, you may take over-the-counter medications such as ibuprofen as directed on the package insert. Ibuprofen is a nonsteroidal anti-inflammatory medication, which works by blocking the production of prostaglandins—a major contributor to pain and cramping during your period. Prostaglandins cause the inflammatory response in the body and might also contribute to symptoms of bloating, nausea, muscle aches, and generalized discomfort. It is important to take ibuprofen at the first sign of your symptoms or a day before the bleeding starts in order to decrease the production of prostaglandins and prevent symptoms from getting worse, says Dr. Roshan.

Nutritional supplements such as vitamin B_6, calcium, vitamin D, and magnesium have been shown to decrease symptoms of PMS. Some studies suggest that these chemicals are paramount for the proper production of brain neurotransmitters such as serotonin and dopamine. As noted previously, there is a direct relationship between serotonin levels and some of the symptoms of PMS, including mood swings, food cravings, depression, and anxiety. Taking supplements is an important PMS intervention as long as you remember that your daily nutrition should include a variety of foods that offer balanced amounts of carbohydrates, proteins, healthy fats, vitamins, minerals, and water. A healthful diet includes an appropriate amount of "healthy fat" (omega-3 fatty acids, for example) essential in maintaining an important balance to counter PMS symptoms. Hormones are produced by the body from sterols. Sterols are fatty substances we get only from a food source. If your diet lacks a proper amount of healthy fat, you might have difficulty producing sufficient amounts of hormones. You may refer to Chapter 5 for a list of food sources of healthy fats.

You might find that reducing your intake of alcohol, caffeine, salt, artificial sweeteners, and refined sugar reduces or eliminates your PMS symptoms. Sodium in salt affects your body by retaining water; therefore, you might feel more bloated and swollen if you consume higher amounts of sodium containing products. Alcohol and coffee are stimulants. As mentioned previously, these put a great burden on your adrenals, which eventually causes an imbalance in cortisol production, leading to progesterone imbalance. Stimulants such as coffee also contribute to fluid retention and irritability. Try to gradually decrease your coffee intake by substituting it with more healthful caffeinated beverages, such as green tea. Some alternative treatments, such as acupuncture, aromatherapy, healing oils, and reflexology, were also found to be helpful in relieving certain PMS symptoms. It is important to find a practitioner in your area who is trained to treat your symptoms. Please ask your primary care practitioner if it is safe for you to use the alternative treatments mentioned above.

Estrogen Dominance

Another common hormonal imbalance seen today is estrogen dominance, which is caused by an imbalance involving estrogen and progesterone; specifically, a relatively low or deficient amount of progesterone in relationship to estrogen. Estrogen dominance was first introduced by Dr. John Lee in his book about natural progesterone. He suggested that a majority of symptoms experienced by women during the premenopausal and menopausal years are caused by an imbalance of estrogen and progesterone levels. In reality, this is not as simple as it sounds.

Let's take a look at what exactly happens, and why our perfectly balanced ovaries become imbalanced. As we age (and what I'm about to mention may occur up to 15 years before we actually enter menopause), we approach the premenopausal years. During this premenopausal time, our progesterone production declines, while estrogen production remains the same or increases. Due to this fact, estrogen becomes a predominant hormone in the body, and without proper counterbalancing of progesterone may cause a list of symptoms, including swollen, tender breasts, impatience and irritability, irregular periods, decreased libido and sex drive, fluid retention, stomach cramps before the onset of menses, fatigue, weight gain, hypoglycemia, mood swings, and depression. Prolonged elevated estrogen levels throughout the years could result in fibrocystic breast disease, polycystic ovarian syndrome (PCOS), endometriosis, endometrial polyps, PMS, uterine fibroids, and breast cancer. In recent years, estrogen dominance is also being documented in the younger female population during their early teenage years. This is not menopause; their progesterone production is still normal. Unfortunately, other external factors also contribute to estrogen dominance. Recent studies note that estrogen dominance may also develop from exposure of the body to external chemicals called *Xenoestrogens.*

What are xenoestrogens, and why haven't we heard of them before? Xenoestrogens are fake or artificial estrogen-like chemicals, which, when entered in the body, tend to mimic estrogen by blocking or binding themselves to estrogen receptor sites, ultimately causing an imbalance of estrogen. Xenoestrogens are chemicals found in products such as phthalates and pesticides. Other chemicals that may have estrogenic effects are hormonal residues found in dairy and meat products. Xenoestrogens accumulate in the body since they are stored in our fat cells. This means it can take the body a long time to get rid of them.

Below is the list of most common products with xenoestrogen chemicals:

Skincare
- 4-Methylbenzylidene camphor (4-MBC) (sunscreen lotions)
- Parabens
- Benzophenone (sunscreen lotions)

Industrial Products and Plastics
- Bisphenol A
- Phthalates (plasticizers)
- DEHP (plasticizer for PVC)
- Polybrominated biphenyl ethers (PBDEs)
- Polychlorinated biphenyls (PCBs)

Food
- Erythrosine / FD&C Red No. 3
- Phenosulfothiazine (a red dye)
- Butylated hydroxyanisole / BHA (food preservative)

Household Chemicals

- Atrazine (weed killer)
- Lindane / gamma-hexachlorocyclohexane (insecticide, used to treat lice and scabies)
- Methoxychlor (insecticide)
- Chlorine and chlorine by-products
- Ethinylestradiol (combined oral contraceptive pill)
- Metalloestrogens (a class of inorganic xenoestrogens)
- Alkylphenol (surfactant used in cleaning detergents)

What Can I Do To Avoid Estrogen Dominance?

As discussed previously, all our glands and the hormones they produce are interconnected. In previous chapters, we discussed the connection between the adrenal gland and thyroid; this chapter shows us that there is a connection between the ovaries and the adrenal gland. But there is also a connection between the ovaries and the thyroid gland as well.

When progesterone levels drop in response to elevated cortisol levels, an imbalance of estrogen (estrogen dominance) blocks the action of the thyroid hormone. As a result, you might suffer from symptoms of hypothyroid disease despite the fact that thyroid hormones in the bloodstream are normal. In order to balance your hormones, it is important to look at the whole picture and work on balancing adrenal, thyroid, and ovarian hormones. For instance, we can't treat the adrenals if we ignore the thyroid or ovaries. So, if we would like to balance the ovaries and avoid estrogen dominance, it is important to address the adrenals and thyroid function as well. Your first step in preventing estrogen dominance is to find a health care practitioner in your area who is trained to diagnose and treat imbalances in adrenal, thyroid, and ovarian hormones.

As discussed in previous chapters, saliva and blood levels will need to be checked to find out what hormonal imbalance is causing your symptoms.

Each body is unique, so there is no single magical pill to balance our hormones. Your practitioner might recommend that you take an herbal supplement, a bio-identical hormone, or a combination of both to help you reestablish hormonal balance. To be effective, you will have to actively participate in your rebalancing journey. You will need an individual approach, and the success of treatment will depend on your ability to change your lifestyle, including your diet, exercise, sleep, and environment.

Your diet will need to include food high in fiber. Estrogen is eliminated partially through our gastrointestinal tract; thus, encouraging frequent bowel movements (not diarrhea, but well-formed stool) serve to increase the elimination of estrogen and prevent its reabsorption. Exercising routinely and maintaining a healthy body weight is another way to decrease estrogen levels in your body.

As mentioned, estrogen is stored in your fat cells. Losing weight and having less fat will decrease your estrogen levels. Switching to organically grown foods will decrease your exposure to xenoestrogens such as pesticides, antibiotics, and growth hormones. The elimination of unhealthy saturated fats, refined sugars, products with artificial sweeteners, and food flavors is also important. It would be overwhelmingly complex to attempt to implement these changes all at once. The "take-away" from this chapter would be to realize that no matter what treatment you are recommended or which herbal or hormonal supplement you are prescribed, to facilitate a healthy, healing journey, your lifestyle must begin to change.

What would the road to recovery and rebalancing look like without lifestyle changes? This is an excellent place to begin. Let's say you are prescribed a bioidentical progesterone supplement to balance your estrogen. Without a lifestyle adjustment, your body might start converting that supplemental progesterone back to estrogen, causing you more symptoms instead of relieving them. One step at the time is all that is necessary in order to begin to implement these changes. Maintaining a healthy life is not a quick fix but rather a lifelong journey. Nelson Mandela said, "*It always seems impossible until it's done.*" This book provides you with a lot of information on how to implement lifestyle changes easily into your daily routine.

Chapter 4

WHY AM I SO TIRED? CHRONIC FATIGUE SYNDROME-MYTH OR REALITY?

"Our fatigue is often caused not by work, but by worry, frustration and resentment" Dale Carnegie

Do you feel tired all or most of the time? A lot of women do, and they often believe it is related to demanding work or family responsibilities. Before you blame your busy lifestyle for your fatigue, let's learn more about what causes chronic fatigue; then we will be able to assess if your symptoms are related to a sporadic lack of rest or to something that requires a more complex intervention. Do you feel exhausted in the morning even after a good night's sleep (at least 7 straight hours)? Do you wake up energized and ready to start the day, or do you often need to drag yourself out from under the covers wishing you could crawl right back in? If you feel tired after sleeping 7–8 or more hours at night, you are not alone. Recent research suggests that 1 in 5 women feel unusually tired, and 1 in 10 have prolonged and debilitating fatigue. This is often caused by an obvious or relatively minor, easy-to-fix problem; however, it may be the sign of a more serious condition such as chronic fatigue syndrome (CFS) or its painful cousin fibromyalgia. These two conditions are often present simultaneously and have overlapping symptoms.

The concept of "chronic fatigue syndrome"(CFS) has only appeared recently in medicine—within the past 20 years. Since its recognition, each year, more cases of this condition are reported—especially in those who live and/or work in developed and industrialized cities. Recently, this problem has become a global epidemic. The appearance of CFS is directly correlated with the sharp acceleration of life's rhythm, increasingly burdensome mental and psychological stress, as well as deteriorating environmental conditions. Statistics show that women, mostly "type A" overachievers, are more susceptible to this condition than are men. CFS is not to be confused with simple tiredness, which serves to alert us that we need to rest. Chronic fatigue syndrome is not a condition that is the result of the occasional lack of sleep; but rather, unfounded, pronounced, debilitating body fatigue that does not go away after adequate rest and prevents the patient from performing activities of daily living. When symptoms of chronic fatigue accumulate, the syndrome becomes quite unbearable. CFS is not a whim or a fantasy and is most certainly NOT "all in your head." It is a serious illness that requires medical attention.

Symptoms of Chronic Fatigue Syndrome

The most common symptoms of CFS are fatigue coupled with severe insomnia or non-restorative sleep, post-exertional weakness, and cognitive dysfunction, often called "brain fog." Orthostatic intolerance—defined as the worsening of symptoms when standing—is also common. Other symptoms of CFS might include the following:

- Sinus problems
- Irritable bowel syndrome
- Weight gain
- Irritability when hungry
- Unexplained muscle pain

- Joint pain without redness or swelling
- Unrefreshing sleep
- Significant impairment of short-term memory or concentration
- Headaches of a new type, pattern, or severity
- Tender cervical or axillary lymph nodes
- Sore throat that is frequent or recurring

Sometimes CFS is difficult to diagnose because its symptoms are similar to those of many other diseases. Before settling on CFS as a diagnosis, other medical conditions associated with fatigue must be ruled out by your health care provider after diagnostic tests have been performed.

Causes of Chronic Fatigue Syndrome

A variety of triggers for chronic fatigue syndrome includes the following:

Sudden Onset

- Postinfectious (e.g. viral, antibiotic sensitive infections, and parasites)
- Postpartum/ after delivery

Gradual Onset:

- Prolonged or frequent emotional and physical stress
- Secondary to autoimmune illnesses (e.g. lupus, MS, and rheumatoid arthritis)
- Fungal infections/Candida
- Hormonal deficiencies (or excess), including thyroid, adrenal, and reproductive
- Toxin exposures (including lead and pesticides)

- A prolonged absence of sun exposure; for instance, during the winter leading to a shortage of "happiness hormone" —serotonin.

- Diseases of the cardiovascular system (atherosclerosis, hypertension and hypotension, anemia)

- Infectious diseases (tuberculosis, Chlamydia, chronic viral infections, and others)

- Cancer, diseases of the nervous system, various functional disorders, and obesity

Research conducted by Harvard University noted that people suffering from chronic fatigue had increased blood levels of melatonin—a hormone produced in the pineal gland that affects the daily biorhythms of the body. Fortunately, most often the fatigue represents a functional disorder rather than a terrible disease. This means as a symptom, the fatigue might be able to be addressed and fixed with a variety of known interventions. Nonetheless, it must be addressed after it is properly diagnosed so we can understand how to deal with it. Fatigue may result from an impairment of blood supply to the brain and peripheral nervous system. Left unaddressed, this results in impairment of the metabolism in our body cells, which lack nutrients, energy, vitamins, and minerals and decreases their ability to function properly. As a result of biochemical processes, we experience an accumulation of cellular waste, built up toxins, and neurotransmitter imbalances that interfere with nerve impulses to and from the brain. All of the factors mentioned above could cause memory impairment, decreased perception, lethargy, and sluggishness. The immune system becomes stressed as a result. This makes the affected person prone to infections from bacteria, viruses, and fungi since a depressed immune system may fail to prevent colds, flu, and other infections.

Treatment of Chronic Fatigue Syndrome

The good news is that CFS is not a deadly disease. Most women recover from it with proper treatment, while others improve tremendously by learning to nurture their bodies from the inside out. Many underlying issues that need to be addressed—from lack of sleep and poor dietary choices to covert infection by viruses or bacteria. In 2013, Dr. Jacob Teitelbaum published an excellent book on chronic fatigue syndrome and fibromyalgia entitled *The Fatigue and Fibromyalgia Solution*. In his book, Dr. Teitelbaum offers a natural treatment approach called the **SHINE** protocol, where he asks readers to address *Sleep, Hormonal imbalances, Infections, Nutrition, and Exercise as able*. A free "Energy Analysis Program" is available at www.endfatigue.com and can be used to help analyze your symptoms in order to determine what factors are contributing to your fatigue. It additionally offers recommendations to help you and your physician optimize your energy.

Sleep

Most women with CFS complain of non-refreshing sleep as a prime concern. If you are one of these women, in order to give your muscles and nervous system a chance to heal, you will need to investigate the reasons for your sleep problems. It is important to discuss with your health care provider your sleep hygiene, causes of insomnia, dos and don'ts of a proper sleep routine, as well as natural methods to help you sleep better. Read more about sleep issues and their treatments in chapter 7 of this book. If you suspect deeper sleep problems such as apnea, consider a visit to a sleep specialist; do not attempt to treat yourself at home.

Hormonal and Adrenal Balance

As discussed previously, hormonal imbalances may be a direct cause of CFS, so balancing your adrenal, thyroid, and ovarian hormones can make a huge difference in treating your symptoms. For information related to testing and treatment for hormonal imbalances, refer to the previous chapters where these issues are addressed.

Infections

The Epstein-Barr virus (EBV) and Lyme disease are two of the most common illnesses seen in association with fibromyalgia and chronic fatigue syndrome. Infection with yeast, parasites, enteroviruses, and other bacteria may also cause CFS. Talk to your health care provider about being tested for these infections so that you can be properly diagnosed and treated.

Nutrition

Proper nutrition is an important aspect of any CFS treatment protocol. In order to heal, your body needs to be provided with whole, fresh foods, such as fruits, vegetables, high-quality fats, and protein (in their natural form—free of preservatives and pesticides, ideally organically grown). High quality vitamin and mineral supplements along with mercury-free fish oil and probiotics help speed the recovery process. It is also important to be aware of any food sensitivities or intolerances you may have since these might be a direct cause of or exacerbate CFS symptoms. Substances such as gluten, sugar, artificial sweeteners, and preservatives are common sources of food allergies. Please consider eliminating these from your diet to see if it makes a difference for you. If you are sensitive, elimination of the foods that irritate your body will notably reduce your CFS symptoms.

Exercise

Exercise is an important part of a healthy lifestyle. Unfortunately, due to body pain and fatigue, women with CFS often adopt a sedentary lifestyle. Incorporating an appropriate exercise regimen should be done gradually, especially for women with CFS.

If exercise has not been part of your regular routine for several months or more begin by starting with easy-stride walking for short periods of time, then gradually increase to a more brisk pace as tolerated. Once the treatment of CFS shows positive results and symptoms decrease, more active forms of exercise such as yoga, Pilates, and aquatic fitness programs may be safely incorporated into your daily exercise routine.

Other factors to consider as we treat CFS include your mind and your emotional health. In treating CFS, it is important to address the mind and body connection. Constant emotional stress drains adrenal reserves and puts stress on hormonal regulation. Hormonal imbalances, as discussed previously, also have a strong impact on CFS. Women with CFS often benefit from psychological counseling, emotional support, and guidance. Breathing exercises, Tai Chi, Qi Gong, and mindfulness meditation are also excellent options to decrease anxiety and help deal with the stress associated with symptoms of CFS.

Treatment of CFS should focus on normalizing the body's energy balance with specific attention on restoring balance in both the parasympathetic and sympathetic nervous systems (the activation and inhibition processes in the body). To do this, various herbal supplements may be used to improve the flow of nerve impulses and the overall nervous system. You may ask your health care provider about the use of certain vitamins, such as B complex, and the role these vitamins play in nerve repair.

It is also valuable to target the nervous system's bioactive points through acupuncture, acupressure, as well as other types of physical therapy throughout the course of treatment. To prevent chronic fatigue syndrome, or at least reduce chances of the extreme negative impact of symptoms, follow a well-balanced diet, try to ensure you get enough quality sleep at night, and exercise regularly. While we can't avoid stress entirely, learning how to minimize the negative impact on our mind, body, and soul from the stress of daily life is essential. We can do this by learning how to manage time and to draw healthy boundaries in relationships to avoid toxicity that is not only unnecessary for us but can actually be destructive to our health.

One example of how to draw healthy boundaries is by asking others to reduce their demands on you and by learning to say "no" to things that feel bad. You are entitled to define your own personal space—mind, body, and soul. Regularly listening to music for relaxation or practicing yoga poses with simple breathing techniques have a calming effect on women suffering with CFS.

Overcoming chronic fatigue is an attainable goal for every woman. Treat yourself well; rationally allocate your time; let yourself relax; try to count your blessings; appreciate your life; practice focusing on the positive aspects in everything, and permit chronic fatigue syndrome to become an experience of the past.

Chapter 5

LET FOOD BE YOUR MEDICINE

"Let food be thy medicine and medicine be thy food." Hippocrates, 460 BC

Eating healthfully is very rewarding but can be confusing to do when there is so much conflicting information available. Fad diets that are tempting and promise quick fixes to our weight; the newest health craze claiming their diet is the only one everyone should follow; prepackaged meals and protein shakes with supplements promising the perfect balance of nutrients and calories flood both bookshelves and social media sites and often times with a hefty price tag. It is so confusing; which one of them is right? Which one should you follow? The table below lists common myths and truths about healthy eating:

Myths Surrounding Healthy Eating	The Truth Surrounding Healthy Eating
Needing to follow strict nutritional philosophies to eat well	Becoming as healthy as possible and having more energy
Have to focus on what I should not eat and restrict myself at every turn	Feeling great and embracing real wholesome foods
Needing to become unrealistically thin	Eating more of what is healthy and less of what is not
Needing to deprive myself of the foods I love	Eating the foods I love with some adjustments

We are all different. We have unique bodies and constitutions, and there is probably no one diet that is right for everyone. So the question to ask is, is it possible to eat healthy and enjoy the food that you love? The good news is you CAN have it all, and to achieve your optimal nutrition status you first need to learn some nutrition basics. The points to keep in mind are that it is very important to follow a balanced diet, and we truly are what we eat. It would be beneficial to focus on choosing foods that are nutrient rich with fewer calories rather than less healthy alternatives. This book provides you with a wealth of information, and all you need to do is use it in a way that works for you. Our bodies are designed to use nutrients to maintain, build, and repair our organs and tissues. It's very important to include 6 nutritional components in our diet on daily basis: carbohydrates, fats, proteins, vitamins, minerals and fluids. Let's take a look at the roles of these nutrients, where we can find them, and the amounts of each recommended in a healthy balanced diet.

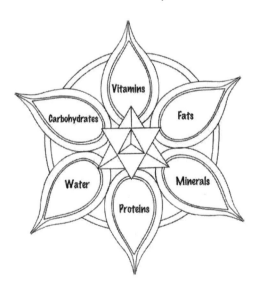

The Healing Flower of Nourishment

Carbohydrates — Energy Source for Your Body

Carbohydrates are very important for bodily functions and metabolism. They are the preferred source of energy for the brain and nervous system, muscle contraction, and other biological work. Carbohydrates supply energy to our organs, enable fat metabolism, and supply dietary fiber. Found in grains, legumes, fruits, vegetables, and dairy products carbohydrates are divided into simple and complex sugars. Simple sugars comprise of glucose, fructose, galactose (monosaccharides), lactose, sucrose, and maltose (disaccharides). Complex sugars are made of longer chains of saccharides known as *polysaccharides*, which form starches. Glucose is the primary source of fuel in our body and when in excess it can be converted to and stored as glycogen. It then may be used to make nonessential amino acids, other essential carbohydrates for specific body compounds such ribose, which is part of RNA and DNA, or be converted to fat and stored in adipose tissue. The liver, pancreas, and insulin all play a role in the conversion, storage, and use of glucose. The liver converts glucose to glycogen to store it for later use. It also takes glycogen out of storage and converts it back to glucose when necessary. The pancreas secretes insulin, which is designed to facilitate the transport of glucose into cells to be used as energy so that the organs and body can function as a working system.

The human body utilizes only glucose for energy, so complex carbohydrates consumed in food need to be broken down to their simplest form: glucose, before they can be used for energy. Some people believe that to increase energy quickly, a large amount of simple sugars should be consumed; however, this is not true. A candy bar, for example, usually has a high carbohydrate and sugar content. Once eaten, it triggers the release of insulin, which quickly lowers the blood sugar and, often times, actually lowers it too much so that the desire for instant energy is the result of low blood sugar just a short time later. This phenomenon is commonly experienced as a sugar high followed by "crashing" an hour or two later. You might ask, "This all sounds very technical. What exactly happens?" Let's see more specifically what happens with glucose metabolism.

All living cells need glucose to function. Insulin is a hormone that is needed to help glucose to enter the cells. Insulin is released once a carbohydrate is ingested, and it acts as a gatekeeper in glucose metabolism. After we ingest carbohydrates, and they enter the bloodstream, insulin alerts the liver to incoming glucose. The liver starts working to metabolize and distribute glucose and use it for energy. Excess glucose is eventually stored in the liver and muscles as glycogen or converted to fat. Insulin also helps glucose to enter the cell thus decreasing blood glucose levels. When you eat simple carbohydrates such as sucrose (sugar found in candy, soda, juice etc.), they are readily broken down and absorbed by the intestines into the bloodstream. This rapid increase in blood glucose leads to a rapid release of insulin that is needed to help transport the sugar into the cells. Energy is rapidly produced but only lasts for a short period of time. So unless a person combines this intake with a protein source or eats another source of carbohydrates soon after the first high carbohydrate food, a hypoglycemic reaction, including symptoms of decreased concentration, sleepiness, tiredness, and decreased energy, might be experienced. Consuming these rapidly releasing sugars, such as white flour, candy, and juices, could lead to "sugar blues," fluctuations from high energy to an energy crash. It is much healthier to consume complex carbohydrates in order to receive a steady supply of glucose and energy.

Complex carbohydrates have a larger structure than simple carbohydrates and take a longer time to absorb and digest. Starch and fiber are examples of complex carbohydrates. Some common foods containing complex carbohydrates include bread, pasta, some vegetables, and whole grains. Due to the slower absorption of sugars in complex carbohydrates (as compared with the glucose of simple carbohydrates), blood glucose levels increase more slowly and result in a slower   rise in insulin levels. Energy is produced in a steady state as compared with the energy spike caused by simple carbohydrates; and lasts for a longer period of time.

It is very important to eat a balanced meal to avoid constant fluctuating levels of glucose and insulin in your bloodstream. If you continuously consume a high carbohydrate diet, eventually, cells trying to protect themselves from glucose overload and will not respond well to insulin. This is known as "insulin resistance." Excess sugar levels in the bloodstream cause the proteins in the body to malfunction, which may lead to a decrease in the effectiveness of the immune system, may damage blood vessels, and negatively affects connective tissues in the joints.

Another benefit of consuming complex carbohydrates is the fiber content. Fiber is found mainly in plants, certain types of fruits, and in many vegetables. Just a few examples of popular, high fiber foods include green leafy vegetables, celery, carrots, apples, and pears. Insoluble fiber is indigestible, provides almost no calories, and encourages the body to feel full. In this way, overeating may be prevented for people sensitive to their own body signals of feeling satisfied during or after a meal. Fiber helps to regulate digestion and metabolism. It stabilizes blood glucose levels and slows down the absorption of nutrients from the intestines. While insoluble fiber adds bulk to the stool helping food to pass through the stomach and intestines at a faster rate regulating digestion, soluble fiber slows digestion helping one to feel satisfied after a meal; which then may decrease the need for constant grazing throughout the day and helps to regulate blood sugar levels. A high fiber diet also helps the body rid itself of waste and chemicals thus decreasing their ability to damage your system.

Glycemic Index and Glycemic Load

Two values help determine the impact of food on our blood glucose and insulin levels. Briefly, the glycemic index (GI) represents the speed at which a specific food breaks down into glucose, and the glycemic load (GL) is the amount of sugar in each portion of food. Together, they help us to choose which carbohydrates are healthiest for us to eat. Generally speaking, the higher the glycemic index of the food, the faster it will be broken down to simple sugar and the greater its impact on the fluctuation in blood sugar and insulin. The bottom line is that we aim to consume foods with lower glycemic index when concerned about blood sugar fluctuations.

Why avoid high blood glucose (blood sugar) levels and fluctuations? A great question. High blood sugar has a negative effect on our body organs and their functions. Specifically, the longer high blood sugar is sustained, the more likely it is to damage blood vessels, negatively affect joint health and mobility, interfere with the immune system, and cause premature ageing of the body as a whole.

Keep in mind that an important factor in assessing the effect of GI and GL on our body is whether foods are eaten individually or in combination with other foods. Another important factor that I would like to point out is the glycemic index and glycemic load of the food is based on consuming a particular food on it is own. Which means the glycemic index and load of the food could be changed if combined with other products. For example, combining simple carbohydrates with proteins or fats at the same meal slows down glucose conversion thus decreasing rapid absorption and reducing chances of a sugar spike in the bloodstream. This is a good thing. A general recommendation for snacking, for example, is to add a protein such as a handful of nuts or nut butters when reaching for a fruit (which is usually high in GI). Another healthy example is to combine vegetables such as carrots with olive oil or guacamole since these are high in a particular type of fat that greatly decreases the rise of glucose in your bloodstream. To achieve a balance of glucose and insulin in the bloodstream, it is important to always eat a balanced meal. For example, corn is a form of complex sugar, which, if eaten by itself, gets into the bloodstream to stimulate insulin production. A sustained excess of sugar in the blood eventually becomes stored as fat. A meal of corn eaten together with chicken or fish, olive oil, and broccoli is a healthy balanced choice. Why? Because with this combination of foods, absorption and digestion are slowed down, and levels of blood glucose and insulin rise slowly and steadily. The body has a chance to utilize this glucose as energy to rebuild tissues rather than to be immediately stored as fat. While working on your nutrition plan, try to choose foods that are listed in the Low GL and Low GI list. These provide the body with a more steady supply of energy and prevent feelings of lethargy and mood swings.

Sugars to Avoid

All man-made carbohydrates, such as white processed table sugars, high fructose corn syrup, fruit juice with sweeteners and concentrates, maple sugar, brown rice and agave syrups, sodas and sugary drinks, and refined white flour products, are recommended to be avoided. Any products that do not grow in nature and can't be grown, picked, gathered, or milked are considered man-made and should not be included in your nutrition plan.

Another product to avoid in your diet is *"artificial sweeteners,"* which have recently gained a lot of media attention. Names such as **Sweet'N Low, NutraSweet,** and others are probably familiar to you. Artificial sweeteners were first discovered by scientists more than hundred years ago. In our continuing battle to lose weight and decrease obesity, artificial sweeteners seemed like a great alternative to refined sugars;

however, they are not as safe as we originally thought them to be. Recent research studies suggest that artificial sweeteners could cause serious changes to our health. These are possible symptoms linked to artificial sweeteners:

- Headaches
- Dizziness
- Intestinal cramping
- Stomach pain
- Agitation
- Menstrual irregularities

- Skin rashes
- Diarrhea
- Bladder issues
- Muscle aches
- Bloating
- Anxiety

Splenda, the newest artificial sweetener on the market, is made out of sucralose and claims to be safer than those that preceded it. Since it has no real track record—not having been on the market for too many years—the long-term effects of its use are still unknown. A better option would be to choose naturally occurring sweeteners, such as raw, unprocessed honey (as processed honey negatively affects the body in a way similar to high fructose corn syrup), stevia, and coconut sugar. The goal is to use sweeteners in moderation and only when absolutely necessary.

Proteins — Building Blocks for Your Body

Proteins are complex molecules made up of hundreds or thousands of smaller units called amino acids. They play substantial roles in the body and are required for the function, structure, and regulation of the body's tissues and organs.

Proteins serve as storage molecules. For example, iron is stored in the liver with the protein ferritin. Proteins also act as transport molecules. Hemoglobin is a protein that transports oxygen. Proteins are the major component of muscle tissues used for movement. They form antibodies needed for immune protection. Proteins are utilized for mechanical support; skin and bone contain collagen, a fibrous protein. Proteins are an important part of hormones that control growth and cell differentiation. They provide 4 cal/g of energy. Some amino acids can be converted to glucose for energy and fuel; however, if consumed in excess of what the body needs, proteins are converted to fat and stored.

Protein is manufactured by your body utilizing dietary protein consumed and thus needs to be consistently replaced. There are 2 different types of proteins: complete and incomplete.

Complete proteins, those with high biologic value, provide adequate amounts and proportions of all the essential amino acids needed for protein synthesis, which is necessary to support tissue growth and repair. Animal proteins and soy protein are complete proteins.

Incomplete proteins lack adequate amounts of one or more essential amino acids and thus might not be able to function properly in the body. Except for soy and hemp protein, all plants are sources of incomplete proteins. Incomplete proteins need to be consumed in combination with other proteins or a small amount of an animal protein to form a complete protein. Some examples of combined proteins are rice and beans, pea soup and toast, a peanut butter sandwich, and a vegetable omelet. The consumption of a complete protein is recommended for optimal body function for several reasons. Mainly, it is better absorbed and more efficiently utilized, thus smaller amounts are needed for optimal function. All animal products—meat, seafood, poultry, dairy, and eggs— are good sources of complete proteins. For people following vegetarian, vegan or raw food diets, it is important to consume adequate quantities of plant-based proteins in combination with complex carbohydrates or different nuts and seeds to make a complete protein. Soybeans can be used as a source of a complete protein. In general, the body needs approximately 20g of protein per meal or 0.8 g/kg of body weight per day. Twenty grams of proteins is equivalent to approximately 3 eggs; 3–4 ounces of poultry, lean meat, or fish; or one cup of cooked beans. Other good sources of proteins are organic unpasteurized dairy products that are non-GMO, free of antibiotics, hormones, and chemicals. Greek style yogurts contain higher amounts of protein and would be more beneficial for those who are vegetarian or vegan. Vegetable protein sources include grains and legumes, nuts and seeds, certain flower vegetables such as broccoli and cauliflower, and combinations of beans and rice or legumes and rice.

Glorious Fats — Binge or a Scourge?

There are so many conflicting opinions regarding fat consumption. Some scientists recommend only low fat or fat free diets, while others argue in favor of high fat or ketogenic diets. Some claim losing weight can only be achieved by low fat or fat free diets, while others argue that eating fat doesn't make you fat.

So which school of thought is right? Let's first find out what type of fats there are and what their function is.

Functions of fat
- Provide energy: 1 g of fat supplies an average of 9 Calories of energy
- Transport fat- soluble vitamins such as A, K, E, and D
- Supply essential fatty acids
- Protect and support organs and bones, and insulate our body from cold

There are several types of fats. Let's take a look at them.

Lipids include triglycerides (fats and oils), phospholipids (e.g., lecithin), and sterols (e.g., cholesterol).

Triglycerides account for approximately 98% of the lipids in foods and are the major storage form of fat in the body.

Phospholipids are structural components of cell membranes that facilitate the transport of fat-soluble substances across cell membranes; they are widespread but appear in small amounts in the diet.

Sterols are one of three main classes of lipids that include cholesterol, bile acids, sex hormones, the adrenocortical hormones, and vitamin D

LDL cholesterol—Low-density lipoprotein (LDL) cholesterol carries cholesterol from the liver to the tissues. An LDL blood level greater than 130 mg/dL is thought to be a contributing factor in arteriosclerosis. LDL cholesterol is considered a "bad cholesterol." Generally, saturated fats and Trans fats are referred to as bad because they raise LDL cholesterol. Unsaturated fats are referred to as good because they lower LDL cholesterol.

HDL cholesterol—High-density lipoprotein (HDL) cholesterol carries cholesterol molecules from the cells to the liver to be excreted. Considered a "good cholesterol", HDL in levels greater than 35 mg/dL are thought to reduce the risk of heart disease. Exercise, maintaining a desirable weight, and giving up smoking are all ways to increase the HDL levels.

Saturated Fats—In general, animal protein contains more saturated than unsaturated fatty acids. Saturated fats are usually solid at room temperature. Examples include meat, poultry, egg yolks, whole milk, cheeses, cream, butter, chocolate, and coconut and palm oil.

Monounsaturated Fats are mostly available from plant-based sources. Examples include olive oil, canola oil, avocados, and cashew nuts.

Polyunsaturated fats—Foods containing high proportions of polyunsaturated fats are usually soft or oily at room temperature. Examples include cooking oils made from sunflower, sesame seeds, corn or soybeans, or soft margarines with liquid vegetable oil as a major ingredient.

Trans fatty acids are produced through the process of hydrogenation; these are chemically unsaturated fats that function like saturated fat in the body. These are considered the unhealthiest fats available since they tend to raise LDL and total cholesterol levels and lower HDL levels. They also alter various metabolic properties in the body and might cause hardening of the arteries. Major sources of these include baked goods, processed crackers, some peanut butters and restaurant foods.

Essential fatty acids are important components of cell membranes. They function to maintain healthy skin and promote normal growth. They cannot be synthesized in the body and thus must be consumed through food. Linoleic acid (n-6) and alpha-linolenic acid (n-3) are essential fatty acids that cannot be made by the body.

Omega-3 fatty acids help to lower serum triglyceride levels, may lower blood pressure and decrease platelet aggregation, and may also have anti-inflammatory effects. The best sources of n-3 fatty acids are fatty cold-water fish, such as salmon, trout, herring, swordfish, sardines, and mackerel. Walnuts, soybeans, flaxseed, and canola oil are examples of plant sources of omega-3 fatty acid alpha-linolenic acid.

As you can see, fats are important for proper body function. The recommendation from the USDA is that adults consume between 20–35% of calories from fat. (Note: young children require as much as 40% according to current thinking). The secret to maintaining a healthy diet is to choose high quality fats that come from cold-water fish such as salmon and tuna as well as from oils derived from nuts and seeds. Fats that come directly from natural sources are beneficial to us, whereas fats from processed foods are not as helpful and may be harmful to the body.

The way in which we prepare our foods may enhance or take away from the value it provides the body. For example, a meal that includes broiled chicken would be considered a healthier choice than a meal of deep fried chicken. This is because of the added oil combined with the high temperature used to fry. When aiming for healthy meal choices, try to use more basic, natural, healthy sources of fat as often as possible. Cook meats thoroughly (internal temperatures should reach 165 degrees—you can use a meat thermometer to help measure this) and at low temperatures when you can. When preparing foods **other than** meat, fish, or poultry, choose to eat them by steaming, gently baking, or broiling. It is important to avoid charring or burning any food as this also reduces its nutritional value.

To obtain an adequate supply of omega-3, it is recommended that we eat fatty fish at least 3 times a week or take a high quality fish oil supplement on a daily basis. Caution should be used when choosing our fish and supplements since products vary widely. Here are some helpful hints: When eating fish or taking fish oil supplements, please be aware of "wild caught" vs. "farmed" as well as the size of the fish. The larger the fish, the greater the mercury content will be. Examples of high mercury containing fish are swordfish and tuna. Examples of smaller fish are sardines. To be sure you are purchasing wild caught salmon, read the product label. It should clearly state the method of catch.

Flaxseed and organic cold-pressed seed oil blends provide balanced ratios of omega-6 and omega-3 fats. It is important to choose **cold-pressed oils** because they provide the essential fatty acids that are otherwise destroyed by heat and refining processes. Do not choose cold-pressed oils for cooking. They are best used as a drizzle or in dressings.

Cooking with cold-pressed oils is not an option to consider when high temperatures are involved. Olive oil and canola oil may be used at low temperatures; however, they shouldn't be used for sautéed or fried dishes because some of the healthiest ingredients are lost during heating. In Part 4 of this book you are provided with delicious recipes using cold-pressed oils with salads and drizzled on steamed, baked, or water sautéed vegetables.

Animal sources provide us with natural saturated fat; they should be used in moderation and preferably from sources that are organic and free of antibiotics and hormones. (When choosing ingredients for our dish, we aim for *stressed fruits and vegetables* and *happy animal products*). The reason for this is stressed vegetables and fruits represent produce that has to fight off insects on its own—without the aid of insecticides. In so doing, they become healthier for humans to eat. Unhappy animals tend to have higher amounts of hormones that are not healthy for humans to eat.

When choosing animal sources for your meals, aim for skinless poultry and lean cuts of beef, which when eaten in small amounts (4 ounce portions), provide fats, proteins, and some vitamins and minerals that are valuable to your health. Eggs are good sources of omega-3 fatty acids and docosahexaenoic acid (DHA), which is necessary for our brain and nervous system. Remember that fats have a high calorie content—twice as many calories per gram as carbs and proteins. Cooking meat, poultry, and any products from animals should be done at low temperatures to avoid damaging the fatty content.

Trans fatty acids should be avoided. Period. Trans fats are artificially produced and during cooking produce higher amounts of polyphenols under high temperatures. Different oils such as soybean or vegetable oil are chemically processed to be solidified into margarine or shortening. Our bodies recognize and are able to digest and metabolize natural fats but are not able to recognize Trans fats; thus, we don't have an enzyme to metabolize them. This means that when Trans fats are consumed, they end up in the bloodstream and contribute to arterial damage and plaque formation. Trans fats are also responsible for inflammation in the body, storage of intra-abdominal fat, and raising LDL cholesterol while lowering HDL. This is a disaster for anyone who wants to eat healthfully and improve total body function.

Trans fatty acids are added to most packaged foods because they prolong their shelf life. They are not listed on the labels as Trans fats, so you need to look at the small letters on the product to see if it contains hydrogenated or partially hydrogenated vegetable oils. This is your biggest clue. In restaurants, avoid eating fried food, and avoid dishes with pie crust—most pie crusts are prepared with shortening as an ingredient. Shortening is high in Trans fats.

Water Is Life

About 60% of an adult's body weight is water. Every adult loses about 2.5 quarts of water per day by perspiring, urinating, and exhaling. To maintain fluid balance in body cells, lost fluid must be replaced. Water is a large percentage of cellular makeup, and it is one of the blood's essential components. It is necessary for controlling body temperature and is involved in almost every body function. Water aids in the digestion and absorption of nutrients, and it transports nutrients and oxygen to cells. Water serves as a solvent for vitamins, minerals, glucose, and amino acids. Under normal conditions, water intake should equal water output to maintain water balance. If the weather is hot, you are exercising or drinking dehydrating fluids such as coffee and alcohol, you will need to increase your fluid intake to prevent dehydration.

What is the best fluid to drink? Plain water is the healthiest choice. It has no calories, absorbs fast, and helps to regulate many body functions. Other fluids to include in your diet are freshly squeezed juices (mixed with filtered water), soups, and teas. To get the best quality water, if it is possible, get a water purifying system to clean excess chemicals and bacteria from the water. Fluids to avoid are sodas, commercially prepared juices from concentrates, and energy drinks. The consumption of coffee and alcohol are up to each individual; if you must drink these, only drink them in moderation.

WILL A SUPPLEMENT A DAY KEEP THE DOCTOR AWAY?

Vitamins and minerals are a very important part of our diet and should be consumed on a daily basis. The best way to get them is through a nutritious and balanced diet—provided that the foods chosen are able to be absorbed by the body (from the perspective of the body as well as the nutrients contained in the food). For example, if the intestines are inflamed, we might not absorb nutrients as well as when our intestines are calm; further, certain fruits picked before they are ripe might not have as much vitamin C as fruits permitted to ripen on the tree or vine.

Another point to keep in mind is that if produce is grown in depleted soil, the opportunity for it to actually absorb the nutrients is not there; thus, we don't receive the nutrients when we eat the fruit. The debate about the value of organically grown produce is an ongoing issue that this book does not explore as thoroughly as the topic deserves, but you are encouraged to research this debate for yourself so you can come to your own conclusions about which choices you deem most beneficial for your diet.

This brings us back to the question about supplements. They are becoming very popular, and according to some resources, everybody should be getting daily vitamin and mineral supplements. You might ask, "If I am following a balanced and a healthy diet, do I really need supplements?" Well you definitely should not be using supplements as a substitute to a healthy and balanced diet. However, as mentioned in the previous section, it is not always possible to receive adequate amounts of necessary nutrients from the food available to us today as compared with the food that was available 100 years ago.

If the soil where food is grown is depleted, the food won't provide the nutrients to our body. An added factor is transportation of produce. Nutrients get lost when food is transported from the farm to the kitchen because of handling, exposure to varied temperatures on trucks, and even from contact with air. Nutrients are also lost during cooking and processing before it even gets to the store. So taking supplements in moderation is one of the ways we can try to make up for the lost vitamins and minerals needed for optimal body function.

Keep in mind that certain supplements may enhance or block each other, so timing, what we take the supplement with, and medications we take may all play a role in how effective our supplementation might be. Iron absorption is thought to be enhanced by taking it with orange juice. Vitamin C helps the body absorb iron from foods and from iron supplements—so these work well together. For more about how the body absorbs vitamins and minerals and which ones work well together, see the references provided at the end of this chapter.

While you can get all the necessary vitamins and minerals from a supplement, it doesn't include fiber or phytochemicals, which you would get from eating the actual food. Supplements should be used as the word suggests: as a supplement to a healthy diet just to be certain you receive adequate amounts of vitamins and minerals on the days when your foods might not fully provide you with all your nutritional needs. Overdosing on certain supplements could be dangerous and toxic. Let's take a look at the functions of vitamins and minerals and their recommended doses.

Vitamins that occur in the actual food are organic substances that can be converted to other forms and are susceptible to oxidation and destruction. Vitamins are an essential component of a healthy diet. Fat-soluble vitamins include vitamins A, D, E, and K. Because they are stored in liver and adipose tissue, vitamins A, D, E, and K do not need to be consumed daily. Water-soluble vitamins include thiamin, riboflavin, niacin, folate, vitamin B6, vitamin B12, pantothenic acid, biotin, and vitamin C. Water-soluble vitamins are not generally stored in the body, so daily intake is necessary. Foods are the natural sources of vitamins and should supply daily vitamin needs.

Minerals are inorganic substances that cannot be broken down and rearranged in the body. The functions of minerals include maintaining fluid and acid/base balance. They play a key role in nerve cell transmission and muscle contraction. Minerals are actively involved in vitamin, enzyme, and hormone activity. It is important to choose the right supplement, so look for supplements that list 100% daily value (DV) for most of the nutrients listed. Never double or triple the recommended does unless under the care of a health care professional (nutritionist, dietician, or other specialist) since vitamins and minerals are beneficial when taken appropriately but may be toxic if taken carelessly. As mentioned above, water-soluble vitamins are not stored in the body, so it is fine if supplements contain more than 100% DV.

Pay attention to the amounts of fat-soluble vitamins such as Vitamin A and E taken since they could easily cause toxicity if consumed in excess. The results of some research studies suggest that excess vitamin E supplementation, for instance, might increase the risk of developing gastrointestinal cancer and heart failure. Beta-carotene, which is a byproduct of Vitamin A, if taken in excess was shown in some research studies to predispose and individual to a higher risk of developing lung cancer.

Folic acid is a water-soluble B vitamin that is not stored in the body and doesn't cause toxicity; however, recent research has indicated that in high doses, folic acid might increase the risk of developing colon polyps and colon cancer. Calcium supplements could cause kidney stone formation, especially if you are genetically predisposed to stone formations. To avoid kidney stone formation, take your calcium supplement in small doses with food spaced throughout the day, and drink plenty of water. If you have any health conditions, always consult your health care provider before taking any supplements. Be aware that many supplements and herbal products have a tendency to interact with prescription medication. Provide your health care provider with the list of supplements you are taking to avoid complications.

Vitamins Table 1

Vitamin	Where can I get it?	Why do I need it?
Vitamin A (Retinol or Beta-carotene)	Retinol—liver, egg yolks, dairy products, margarine Beta-carotene — dark green and deep yellow fruits and vegetables	Keeps eyes healthy; develops bones; protects linings of respiratory, digestive and urinary tracts; maintains healthy skin and hair. Beta-carotene fights free radicals.
Vitamin B_1 (Thiamine)	Whole grains, cereals and enriched grain products, legumes, organ meats, lean pork, and eggs	Promotes healthy functioning of the nerves, muscles, and heart. Metabolizes carbohydrates
Vitamin B_2 (Riboflavin)	Organ meats, enriched breads and cereals, legumes, almonds, cheese and eggs, meat, fish, and dark green vegetables	Metabolizes carbohydrates, fats, and proteins, produces hormones, and promotes eye and skin health.
Vitamin B_3 (Niacin)	Meat, organ meats, whole grains and cereals, legumes, eggs, milk, green leafy vegetables, and fish	Metabolizes carbohydrates and fats, helps functioning of digestive system, and maintains healthy skin
Vitamin B_5 (Pantothenic Acid)	Organ meats, yeast, raw vegetables, eggs, and dairy products	Produces hormones, and maintains body's immune system
Vitamin B_6 (Pyridoxine)	Whole-grain products, poultry, fish, nuts, meat, fruits, vegetables, eggs, and dairy products	Metabolizes protein, helps produce hemoglobin, promotes functioning of digestive and nervous systems, and maintains healthy skin
Vitamin B_{12} (Cyanocobalamin)	Organ meats; fish, lean meats, poultry, cheese, and eggs	Builds genetic material of cells, and produces blood cells
Vitamin C (Ascorbic Acid)	Fruits and vegetables (especially citrus fruits, tomatoes, peppers, strawberries, and cantaloupe)	Acts as an antioxidant, fights and resists infection, heals wounds, and promotes growth and maintenance of bones, teeth, gums, ligaments, and blood vessels
Vitamin D (Cholecalciferol)	sun exposure is the primary source of vitamin D. Fortified milk, eggs, fish-liver oils, and fatty fish such as herring, mackerel, and salmon	Builds strong bones and teeth, and maintains the nervous system.
Vitamin E (Tocopherol)	Vegetable oils, nuts, wheat germ and whole-wheat products, egg yolks, and green leafy vegetables	Protects the lungs, nervous system, and skeletal muscle; may reduce risk of heart disease by protecting against atherosclerosis
Vitamin B_7 (Biotin)	Oats, organ meats, yeast, and eggs (cooked), whole-wheat products, dairy products, fish, and tomatoes	Metabolizes proteins and carbohydrates; breaks down fatty acids
Vitamin K	Dark green leafy vegetables, eggs, cheese, pork, and liver	Promotes normal blood clotting.
Vitamin B_9 (Folic Acid)	Vegetables (especially dark-green ones), organ meats, whole-wheat products, legumes, and mushrooms	Synthesizes protein and genetic materials; may help prevent some cancers, heart disease, and stroke

Minerals Table 2

Mineral	Where could I get it?	Why do I need it?
Calcium (Ca)	Milk and dairy products, dark-green vegetables, legumes, shellfish, tofu, and calcium-fortified orange juice.	Builds bones and teeth; promotes blood clotting, contraction of muscles, and nerve impulses
Copper (Cu)	Organ meats, shellfish, whole-grain products, legumes and dried fruits	Builds bones, red blood cells, and hemoglobin; metabolizes iron, and maintains connective tissue and blood vessels
Fluoride (F)	Seafood, tea, coffee, and soybeans; sodium fluoride is often added to the water supply to prevent tooth decay.	Promotes bone and tooth formation; prevents tooth decay.
Iodine (I_2)	Saltwater fish, shellfish, sea kelp, and iodized salt.	Helps produce thyroid hormones
Iron (Fe)	Red meat, organ meats, whole-wheat products, shellfish, nuts, dried fruit, and breads and cereals enriched with iron	Helps produce hemoglobin and red blood cells; delivers oxygen to muscles and other body tissues;
Magnesium (Mg)	Legumes, whole-grain cereals, nuts, dark-green vegetables, meat, seafood, and dairy products	Builds bones and teeth and is involved in functioning of muscular and nervous systems
Manganese (Mn)	Tea, green vegetables, legumes, oats, and rice	Involved in reproductive processes, sex hormone formation; essential for normal brain function and bone development
Phosphorus (P)	Meat, fish, eggs, legumes, dairy products, whole wheat, corn, and rice.	Builds bones and teeth
Potassium (K)	Potatoes, dried fruits, bananas, legumes, raw vegetables, avocados, mushrooms, lean meat, milk, and fish	Helps nerves and muscles function; regulates heart's rhythm; regulates bodily fluids
Selenium (Se)	Whole-grain cereals, fish and shellfish, meat, and dairy products	Acts as an antioxidant; helps protect cells and tissues from damage by free radicals
Sodium (Na)	Found naturally in many foods and is added to many prepared foods	Maintains body's fluid balance and is important for nerve function and muscle contraction; controls heart's rhythm
Zinc (Zn)	Shellfish, organ meats, lean red meat, yeast, whole-grain cereals, and legumes	Important for skin health, wound healing, protein metabolism, and energy production

PROBIOTICS — A MILLION FRIENDS IN YOUR GUT

You have probably heard of probiotics. They seem to be mentioned everywhere—from television commercials to advertisements in magazines. They are added to many products, and multiple research studies are being conducted nationally to investigate their benefits.

So what are probiotics, and what is all this hype about? Probiotic literally means "for life" and are naturally occurring bacterial flora in our gastrointestinal tract. We have millions of small organisms living in our gut that help us to digest and absorb food, synthesize vitamins K, B, and A, and maintain our immune function. The appendix is thought to regulate the gut flora, and unfortunately, a majority of us don't have a healthy balance of gut flora for several possible reasons. One might be that the appendix has been removed. Another is that our "good bacteria" have been destroyed by antibiotics, stress, birth control pills, alcohol, or acid blocking medications.

Live culture yogurt supplies the body with certain species of beneficial bacteria. Dairy products and fermented vegetables such as sauerkraut and pickles, some sourdough breads, and fermented soy products also supply probiotics for our gut. Enjoy these foods daily to receive your healthy doses of probiotics (keeping in mind that if you are on a salt restricted diet, you may need to monitor your intake).

Take probiotic supplementation (up to 20 billion is usually recommended) as needed if you are prescribed antibiotics for infections. If you are on an antibiotic, the timing of taking the probiotic supplement should be discussed with your health care provider. Choose probiotics that supply a variety of bacteria including *bifidobacterium* and *lactobacillus acidophilus*. In general, if not on an antibiotic, you may take probiotics before meals twice a day. Choose an enteric-coated variety to prevent the stomach acid from destroying the bacteria.

ANTIOXIDANTS — LITTLE BODYGUARDS OF YOUR CELLS

Perhaps you have heard about antioxidants. This word is often used in advertising and popular science programs, but the definition is not always offered. This chapter will hopefully clarify what antioxidants are and why they are so important.

It is believed that antioxidants are substances that facilitate healing and protection from the inside of our body. It is thought that their impact helps keep us alive longer while protecting our cells so we maintain good health. So, you might ask, "What are these wonderful substances, and what is so special about them?"

The human body constantly produces oxidants or *free radicals*—molecules that have increased chemical activity. Under the influence of adverse factors (poor environmental conditions, poor diet, stress, smoking, alcohol, etc.), excessive amounts of "oxidants" produced begin to destroy otherwise perfectly healthy cells, tissues, and organs. Antioxidants are substances capable of binding and thereby neutralizing free radicals. This means that antioxidants work by preventing those free radicals from damaging cell membranes, speeding up recovery from destruction, and increasing our resistance to infection.

Antioxidants became the center of public attention in the 1990s, when scientists began to realize that free radicals contribute to the early stages of artery-clogging atherosclerosis and can cause cancer, vision loss, and many other chronic diseases. Some studies have shown that people with an inadequate intake of antioxidant-rich fruits and vegetables are at greater risk of developing these chronic diseases than people who consume these foods in large quantities every day. Clinical studies have shown the effects of individual substances, particularly beta-carotene and vitamin E, as a weapon against heart disease, cancer, and other chronic diseases.

What Are Antioxidants, And Where Can I Find Them?

Hundreds, perhaps thousands, of different substances may act as antioxidants. The best known of these are vitamin C, vitamin E, beta-carotene, and other carotenoids with minerals such as selenium and manganese. Other antioxidants include glutathione, coenzyme Q10, lipoic acid, flavonoids, phenols, polyphenols, and phytoestrogens.

Plant foods are a rich source of antioxidants. Antioxidants are most abundant in fruits and vegetables, nuts, whole grains, and certain varieties of meat, poultry, and fish. So if you want to protect your body from free radicals, your diet should contain natural products and be diverse in composition. Eating at least 2 cups of fruit and 2 ½ cups of vegetables every day is a good start for a healthy lifestyle. It is also believed that antioxidants and other protective components of vegetables, legumes, and fruits should be regularly consumed beginning in early childhood in order to be effective. High sources of antioxidants include products such as raisins, pomegranates, blueberries, prunes, blackberries, kale, spinach, and broccoli.

FOOD CRAVINGS — WHERE DO THEY COME FROM?

We have all experienced food cravings at some point in our lives. Certain cravings come during times of stress. Comfort foods are selected to satisfy us at these times. Hunger is a desire for food when the body is low in energy. Some people crave sweets, while others crave salty products, chocolate, or fatty foods. Some scientists suggest that "craving" as an experience is rooted in psychological factors. It is also argued that cravings are actually messages sent by the body to inform us that we need certain nutrients. Other schools of thought hold that cravings are actually important to fight off since the body may crave a food to which it is actually allergic or unfortunately oversensitive.

Women tend to have higher rates of food cravings than do men, especially before and during menstruation. Statistically, women crave more sweet and sugary substances, while men prefer fatty foods, such as barbequed meat and French fries. So what is the reason for food cravings? Is it caused by hunger, emotional needs, or a nutritional deficiency? This chapter will explore these ideas, among others. Remember that we are each individual beings with separate body chemistries. We might experience cravings several times a month, just a few times a year, or not at all. We may crave sweets or chocolate, comfort food, or none of these things. This chapter will help answer some common questions and will hopefully offer helpful hints and tips.

What Drives Hunger?

"Hunger" and "craving" are not the same thing. One could actually have food cravings even when not hungry. The body uses a hormone called *ghrelin* to stimulate the hypothalamus, which in turn stimulates appetite. When we eat food, our fat tissues release a hormone called *leptin*, which controls our feeling "full" or satiated and tells the body we can stop eating. Ghrelin, as a messenger, delivers a message to the hypothalamus that it is time to eat but doesn't specify what to eat. It doesn't ask for a cheesecake or cheeseburger. It just expresses a message that the body needs to eat something. *Anything.* Cravings, however, are more complicated than hunger. They involve the brain differently as they engage a cascade of hormones and possibly involve complex nutritional needs.

What Drives Cravings?

Cravings are often influenced by neurotransmitters in the brain such as serotonin and dopamine. These are two examples of hormones that trigger the experience of pleasure and feeling good. These hormones are released when we eat foods that we love and enjoy. Although it is possible, most people don't generally crave broccoli and spinach. More common food cravings include choices loaded with refined sugar, fat, and salt. This may be because the human body generally feels a rush of euphoria when eating these foods, and the brain, understandably, seeks that experience over and over.

What May Trigger Food Cravings?

Cravings may be triggered by an *insufficient level of dopamine or serotonin.* For instance, when stressed-out or under pressure, the adrenal glands produce cortisol while the brain has a low serotonin level. We start craving comfort or pleasure food such as those high in simple carbohydrates, which if eaten, increase insulin levels in the blood and stimulate the brain to release stored serotonin. We suddenly feel better, our mood improves, and we function well. However, this serotonin rush doesn't last long, and soon after, we generally feel tired or cranky again. If we permit this loop to continue, we then satisfy the craving with more of that same food. We usually crave only foods that we ate and liked before rather than foods we have never heard of. This is because, for most people, food cravings are connected to sensory memories formed in association with those foods. For instance, if you happen to crave an apple pie, specifically, your grandmother's apple pie—the pie you believe is "the best"— this craving is probably related to the positive association you have with the wonderful time you spent with your grandmother or your family while eating her pie. So, in this case, our brain reward system involves our food cravings as a physiological way to trigger familiar pleasures and to increase serotonin levels in the body. In order to minimize the chance of cravings caused by low serotonin levels, it is important to eat a balanced diet so you have all the nutrients your brain needs in order to produce enough serotonin.

When under pressure and experiencing a lot of emotional or physiological stress, your body might develop intense cravings as well. Adrenal glands are responsible for producing cortisol in response to stress. Cortisol regulates sugar metabolism. When your body is under stress, your blood cortisol levels may go up and down, causing the blood glucose levels to fluctuate as well. This often contributes to the energy crashes, tiredness, fatigue symptoms, and food cravings that you might be experiencing. To check your cortisol levels and your adrenal gland functions, you will need to ask your health care practitioner to check your saliva cortisol levels as discussed previously in Chapter 3 of this book. You will also need to focus on how you manage life stressors.

Mastering effective stress management techniques helps us feel more in control and less burdened. While it is not possible to completely avoid all stressful situations in our lives, it is definitely possible to learn to manage all we must deal with. Another way to say this is that it is not how much stress we are exposed to that matters but rather how much of it we permit to affect us. Our reaction to stress plays a much bigger role in its effect on our body. Meditation, breathing exercises, and other stress management techniques might help you deal more effectively with stressful situations and, ultimately, prevent those intense stress-related cravings.

Another common reason for food cravings is *blood sugar dysregulation and cortisol production imbalance.* Many women complain of intense cravings during the afternoon around 3–4 p.m. when they experience what is often referred to as the "afternoon crash." This is thought to be caused by an afternoon drop in levels of blood cortisol and blood sugar. Blood sugar (or glucose) supplies the energy for cells in the body, specifically, for the brain. When blood sugar levels drop, our brain cells—deprived of glucose—send a message to the body to get food. The specification is sadly often for something with lots of simple sugar. The goal, from the brain's perspective, is to quickly raise blood glucose levels. Since sugary foods like cookies, candies, chocolate, and other processed products and drinks raise our blood sugar quickly, we often crave those types of snacks.

To prevent food cravings and mid-afternoon crashes, it is important to keep your blood glucose levels balanced by eating a small meal or snack every 2–3 hours. Preferably, choose your snacks from the more healthy varieties of fruits, vegetables, and proteins. Good choices include combinations of vegetables, proteins, and healthy fats; for example, carrots and hummus, apples with peanut or almond butter, or cucumber or celery with a bean dip.

Another reason to crave salty chips might be that your body is trying to tell you that you are missing some important nutrients. It is believed that craving salty snacks signals that the body might be deficient in minerals such as potassium, calcium, or iron. If you crave chocolate, your body might need a mineral such as magnesium, which raw cacao provides. If you eat chocolate, make sure you eat a good quality dark chocolate made with 75% or higher organic raw cacao, and add other high magnesium containing foods to your diet, such as fish, leafy greens, seeds, and nuts.

Cravings for cheese might be a signal that the body is deficient in fatty acids. Eating more foods such as fish, walnuts, and flaxseeds might prevent fatty acid deficiency and decrease cheese cravings. Craving foods such as steak and other meat containing meals might indicate an iron deficiency. It is not uncommon for women to crave a hamburger during or after menstruation, when iron levels in the blood may be depleted. Increasing your intake of beans, legumes, figs, prunes, and other dried fruits will increase your iron levels and decrease meat cravings.

How else can we prevent food cravings? It is important to consume a balanced diet including healthy fats, proteins, carbohydrates, vitamins, and minerals. Time your meals and snacks every 2–3 hours throughout the day to avoid blood sugar fluctuation and energy crashes. Drink plenty of fluids to keep well hydrated. Learn and practice stress management techniques to avoid draining your adrenal glands and to prevent cortisol dysregulation. But if you do occasionally crave a slice of your favorite grandmother's apple pie, go ahead - call or visit your grandmother if you able to, or organize a family dinner where you can have a great time and, yes, maybe even get that favorite slice of apple pie. Remember, eating comfort foods occasionally with your family is healthy and beneficial for you physically and emotionally, so enjoy it when you have the opportunity.

FOOD SENSITIVITIES, ALLERGIES, AND INTOLERANCES

Food sensitivities, allergies, and intolerances are being mentioned more and more often today. These terms are often used interchangeably and may be quite confusing to many people. Are food allergies the same as food sensitivities? Are food intolerances the same as food allergies? Let's take a look at them each individually.

Food allergies are more serious than intolerances or sensitivities and are toxic reactions to foods or food additives. Allergies usually involve our immune system—the immunoglobulin E (IgE) antibody. An allergic reaction is usually immediate and occurs within several minutes or an hour after exposure to the allergen that was ingested, smelled, or touched. Some people are so allergic to peanuts that even smelling the airborne particles of a bite of a peanut butter sandwich eaten by someone else is enough to set off the allergic response. Symptoms range from mild to severe and may include itching, hives, a runny nose, sneezing, difficulty breathing, wheezing, or the most dangerous of all: anaphylactic shock (a severe and sometimes fatal allergic response), which might require hospitalization. The US Centers for Disease Control report 8 food types that cause 90% of food allergies: cow's milk, hen's eggs, peanuts, soy foods, wheat, fish, crustacean shellfish (such as shrimp, prawns, lobster, and crab), and tree nuts (such as almonds, cashews, walnuts, pecans, pistachios, Brazil nuts, hazelnuts, and chestnuts).

Food intolerances mostly occur when there is a lack of production of a particular enzyme, and the individual is not able to digest a particular food. This might cause symptoms several hours after the food has been ingested. Lactose intolerance and celiac disease are two examples of food intolerances. Ingesting foods that irritate the individual might cause a variety of symptoms that are not life threatening but are nonetheless very uncomfortable. Lactose intolerance is caused by a lack of the digestive enzyme called lactase, which is needed to break down and digest lactose, a sugar found in dairy products. After the ingestion of dairy products, a lactose intolerant person might complain of abdominal cramping, bloating, gas, and diarrhea.

Sensitivity vs. Disease The terms "gluten sensitivity" and "celiac disease" are often used interchangeably, but they are not the same. Gluten is a protein found in wheat and other grains such as rye and barley. *People with celiac disease have a multisystem autoimmune disease,* which causes changes in liver function, the digestive tract, and other organ systems in the body. The ingestion of gluten causes an immune response that attacks and damages the wall of the small intestines. As a result, nutrient absorption decreases. The long-term effects of celiac disease include conditions such as anemia, osteoporosis, multiple sclerosis, migraines, intestinal cancers, infertility, and miscarriages. Treatment for this disorder is to follow a strict gluten free diet.

A person with gluten *sensitivity*, on the other hand, might exhibit similar symptoms as one who suffers from celiac disease; however, when tested, will not show positive for antibodies in the bloodstream and will not show intestinal damage as seen in persons with celiac disease. Additionally, people with gluten sensitivity might exhibit non-GI symptoms such as joint pain, headaches, and numbness in the extremities, generalized malaise, brain fog, and loss of concentration. Symptoms might appear days after the ingestion of gluten containing products. Treatment for this condition is following an elimination diet discussed below.

Food sensitivities are called "hidden" or "delayed" allergic reactions, which are considered a more subtle reaction to foods. As mentioned above, they might occur several days after the suspected food has been ingested; thus, it is often difficult to make the connection that the symptoms are related to a particular food. These reactions are immunoglobulin G (IgG) mediated and might cause generalized symptoms including but not limited to fatigue, migraine headaches, irritable bowel syndrome, sleep disturbances, joint pain, nausea, or acid reflux.

Recent research indicates there is a very close relationship between the gastrointestinal tract and our immune system. Our GI tract is surrounded by immune system cells that have a direct relationship with our gut flora. Thousands of different types of bacteria living in our gut have a direct relationship with our immune system and support our digestion, detoxification, nutrient synthesis, and control our inflammatory responses to food. The development of different food sensitivities might be directly related to an imbalance in our intestinal flora (good bacteria), which might contribute to chronic gut inflammation. Constant exposure to inflammatory food eventually causes chronic inflammation throughout the body, and this reaction is responsible for causing a long list of systemic symptoms. This silent inflammation is suspected to be a major contributing factor in most chronic diseases such as Alzheimer's, heart disease, cancer, obesity, diabetes, mood disorders, and autoimmune diseases. Common foods that cause sensitivities include highly processed foods, refined sugars, refined flours, artificial sweeteners, various food additives and preservatives, as well as products containing wheat and gluten.

Which Food I Should Avoid?

Food sensitivities and allergies are very individual, and you know your body better than anyone else does. Knowing yourself is important in order to figure out which foods may be toxic and which foods may be best for you. If you know, for example, that after eating a particular food, you feel a particular way, you can learn what experiences, reactions, moods, and symptoms each food causes.

Keeping a daily diary of foods, symptoms, and moods would be helpful in figuring out what is good for you and what you may need to avoid. If a certain food causes you to have a severe allergic reaction, the easiest solution is to avoid this type of food and to read the labels on all products to avoid accidental exposure to it. If you suspect you have a food intolerance or sensitivity but are not sure which food might be causing all the symptoms, ask your health care practitioner to test you for food allergies. A simple blood test can check your IgE levels after ingesting a particular food and confirm your allergy to it.

Food sensitivities or IgG mediated reactions are more complex to detect. There are several ways to be tested, and one of them is the blood test called the ALCAT—antigen leucocyte antibody test. This blood test measures your body response to different dietary substances and may be used as a tool to help to adjust your diet and decrease inflammatory responses in your body. This test is not available in some states and might not be reimbursed by certain health insurance companies.

Another option involves a combination of keeping the food diary mentioned above with an elimination diet approach. This is a relatively inexpensive test method, but it requires consistency and some work on your part. Start to eliminate a type of food that you suspect might be causing your symptoms. For example, you might decide to avoid refined sugar or wheat, for 2–3 weeks, constantly monitoring your progress and your symptoms. After 3 weeks, slowly reintroduce the eliminated food, and monitor your reaction to it. If you notice changes in your symptoms, it might be an indication that you are sensitive to this particular food and should avoid it in the future. If you suspect multiple food sensitivities or are not able to tolerate the elimination diet, find a practitioner who is trained in diagnosing food sensitivities to help you to successfully eliminate these products from your diet.

Chapter 6

WHAT DIET IS BEST FOR YOU?

"Your diet is a bank account; good food choices are good investments."
Bethanny Frankel

Our bodies are unique. This means that we each have our own individual biological responses to different foods we consume, including the ways in which we metabolize these foods. With these points in mind, we need to individualize our approach in choosing and balancing foods in our diet. It seems that every day we hear of a new diet emerging, with claims that it is the best choice for everyone. It is logical for people to rush to try this perfect diet; some really benefit from it and feel terrific, while others feel worse than before. Sadly, there is no single diet appropriate for all. For example, some do well on a strict vegetarian diet, while others do not. A diet that works for you might not work as well or at all for your husband, partner, sibling, or children. Why not? What is missing, and how should you choose a perfect diet for you and your family?

I am afraid that there is no single correct answer to these questions. You and only you know what the best food for you is. You can experiment with different types of diets, see how you feel, then choose the one that gives you energy and helps you feel great. In this chapter, I will cover a few popular diets. I will review their basic philosophy, and you can then decide which ones to try to see which, if any, can work for you and each member of your family. However, before I introduce types of diets to you, I would like to talk about important characteristics that make you unique, such as gender, culture, and age, which you should consider while choosing your diet.

Does Gender Affect What You Eat?

Men and women do eat differently; this topic was researched at length, with different theories proposed as to why women eat differently from men. Men mostly prefer high protein sources of food, such as beef, while women prefer fruits, vegetables, and sweets, such as chocolate and cupcakes. Some studies suggest that men have more muscle mass and thus require more protein in their bodies, which may help explain their preference for high protein containing foods.

Another explanation suggests differences in taste bud sensitivity. Men, according to research, have a lower sensitivity to bitterness, while women are more sensitive to bitter tastes and thus prefer sweets. It might also be a socially acceptable norm for men to eat bigger portions of steak, which might be linked to their image of masculinity and strength. Women in our society, on the other hand, have greater concerns regarding their weight control and thus tend to select low fat foods, including fruits and vegetables. Regardless of the reason, when selecting a diet for yourself and your family, it is important to take these differences into consideration.

Does Age Affect What You Eat?

Age may be another factor in determining what foods to eat. Nutritional needs change throughout our life span, and adults have different nutritional needs as compared with those of children or older adults. For instance, children and teenagers, who are in the process of developing and growing rapidly, require higher and more nutritionally dense foods. People in their sixth decade of life and older have slower metabolisms and tissue regeneration; therefore, older adults may need to consume smaller amounts and different types of foods—unless they are extraordinary athletes and follow unusually energetic exercise routines more common to younger bodies. A body with a degenerative disease also experiences unique dietary needs.

Does Culture Affect What You Eat?

Culture is another important factor to consider when choosing healthy meals. Our food choices are greatly affected by our culture, both consciously and subconsciously. Culture determines the choice, timing, combination, and preparation of food since it defines what is and what is not acceptable to us. Food preparation and consumption are symbolic on multiple levels, including mind, body and soul—all of which are affected by culture. Culture is not instinctive; it is learned and passed from generation to generation. Culture is not static; it is able to adapt and change. Attempting to change a diet without regarding personal culture and tradition is a common mistake. Respect and awareness are key to success. Working within each person's preferences on all levels facilitates a successful journey to healthful diet planning. Slowly incorporating healthy choices while reducing less healthy ones may take time, but the results guide us as increasing wellness and reduced symptoms positively influence our healthful choices. Dietary changes should not be drastic; rather, they should be small steps in a long-term process so the mind, body, and soul have time to adjust.

Another aspect to consider is your body's reaction to new foods consumed. If certain food groups have been consumed for generation in your culture, you likely have the ability to digest them properly. Your body may be accustomed to a type of food and might crave it on occasion. A note of caution is offered by Dr. Nancy Iankowitz, Director of Holistic and Integrative Healing, whose practice specializes in stress management and gastrointestinal health: "Just because a particular food might be customarily or traditionally consumed by your family does not mean it is actually good for your system." A self-test may include eliminating a particular food to notice whether your bowel pattern changes. For example, if you always considered it usual to have gas, constipation, or loose stool, consider eliminating different foods or changing around the order of their consumption to see if your gastrointestinal patterns improve. Gas, bloating, constipation, and diarrhea are not health expressions but are indicative of intolerance. An example of a food intolerance related to genetics would be "lactose intolerance," which is more predominant in people from certain cultures and ethnic backgrounds. For instance, according to statistical data, people from Asian cultures have a higher incidence of lactose intolerance as compared with others, and their diets reflect that phenomenon since few dairy products are consumed as part of their daily food intake.

Cultures also determine our health beliefs about food and its relationship to body shape and constitution. Different cultures have used a variety of foods as healing remedies for common illnesses for generations. Also, healthy body image is represented differently in various cultures; in some cultures, a certain percentage of body fat is considered "overweight" while in other cultures, that same percentage is considered a sign of good health and well-being. Certain cultures view a lean body as one that suggests wellness, fitness, and beauty, while other cultures view that same body as indicative of sickness.

If you happen to be from a culture that strives for a greater percentage of body fat than what you personally strive for, changing your diet to lose weight might become a difficult endeavor. If you secretly believe it is beautiful or healthier to have that higher percentage of body fat or if family pressure has a great impact on your personal goals, your efforts will certainly be undercut. Therefore, in order to be successful in changing your food choices to a healthier, balanced diet, you might first benefit from honest self-reflection.

Below, you will find information on different types of diets; the list is very short given the limited space in this book. Consider this list a starting point. You may choose one of the diets below just to see if it works for you and your family. Diets such as these offer structure and guidelines that are easy to follow. In addition, there are recipes and a shopping list to help guide you. Feel free to do what makes sense to you—no need to strictly follow a particular diet to begin your healing journey. You may choose to take some ideas and slowly adjust a few food choices at a time as you notice great results. The choice is yours; decide what will work best for you and your lifestyle. *A word of caution:* Before adopting a new diet, check with your health care provider to see if one particular diet might be better for you than another would.

Vegetarian Diets

The vegetarian diet dates far back, with roots in ancient India and ancient Greece. Vegetarianism is more than just a diet. It is a way of living that follows an idea of animal nonviolence, which is called *Ahisma* in India and includes avoidance of consuming for food or utilizing in life any products from animal sources. There are different types of vegetarian diets:

- **Vegan** — Avoids all foods of animal origin
- **Ovo-Vegetarian** — Excludes all animal flesh and milk but consumes eggs
- **Lacto-Vegetarian** — Excludes all animal flesh and eggs but consumes milk
- **Lacto-Ovo Vegetarian** — Avoids all animal flesh but consumes eggs and milk
- **Pesco-Vegetarian** — Avoids red meat and fowl but consumes fish and seafood

- **Semi or Partial-Vegetarian** — Uses some milk products, eggs, poultry, and fish, but consumes primarily plant-based foods.

All forms of vegetarian diets are high in fruit and vegetable content and low in saturated fat and animal protein. They're also high in antioxidants, vitamins C, E, and phytochemicals. Becoming vegetarian is more complex than simply eliminating animal food. It is important to make sure to balance a vegetarian diet to include all major food components, such as carbohydrates, proteins, and healthy fats. If a vegetarian diet is not balanced properly, you might become deficient in important vitamins and minerals such as iron, vitamin B_{12}, calcium and vitamin D.

High Protein Diets

High protein diets focus on decreasing carbohydrate consumption by obtaining calories and nutrients from protein and fats. The most popular high protein diet is a well-known Atkins diet. The main idea of the diet is to consume less carbohydrates, which will force the body to burn it is own fat for energy and cause weight loss. It is a form of ketogenic diet where ketones are produced during the process of fat breakdown. This diet is designed to work in phases where different foods are eliminated throughout the phase.

High protein and high fat intake increases satiety level, so people on this diet consume fewer calories and are more successful in losing weight. People following this diet get the wrong impression of the Atkins diet, which promotes unlimited amounts of fatty meats and dairy products. It is important to keep in mind that choosing healthier versions of proteins and fats will prevent long-term problems such as diabetes and cardiovascular disease. If not balanced properly, this diet might also cause deficiencies in fiber and some vitamins and minerals.

High Carbohydrate Diets

One of the most popular high-carbohydrate diets is the Dr. Dean Ornish diet. This diet focuses on eating low-fat, low-protein, and high-carbohydrate diet food and avoids eating meats. The Dr. Ornish diet is designed specifically for people at risk or with history of cardiovascular disease. His diet is plant based and restricts fat consumption thus decreasing arterial aging and atherosclerotic plaque formation. Research studies conducted confirmed benefits of the Dr. Ornish diet and his lifestyle recommendations for cardiovascular health, and now some insurance companies actually reimburse patients following this particular regimen.

Dr. Ornish also recommends changes in lifestyle to compliment his diet principles such as to stop smoking, increase exercise, and reduce stress. Due to the low fat content of the diet, it might predispose people to deficiencies of fat-soluble vitamins if not balanced properly. To balance this diet, it might be beneficial to add a small variety of healthy fats such as nuts, avocados, olive oil, and fish.

Mediterranean Diet

The Mediterranean diet is becoming more popular lately due to claims that it has a profound ability to prevent cardiovascular disorders such as heart attack and stroke. Researches who investigated different diets noticed that people living in the countries of Mediterranean region, such as Greece, Italy, France and Spain, have lower rates of heart disease. The general diet principles of people from these countries includes the high consumption of fruits, vegetables, whole grains, beans, olives, olive oil, nuts, and seeds, as well as a moderate intake of wine and lean meats and low intake of processed foods. Lifestyle factors such as increased physical activity and enjoying meals with a social support system are also part of the Mediterranean way of life.

A large percentage of total fat in the Mediterranean diet is from monounsaturated fat, which is largely responsible for the reduction in heart disease because it does not raise cholesterol levels the way saturated and Trans fats do. Other benefits of the Mediterranean diet include a high concentration of cancer-fighting antioxidants because of the emphasis on fruit and vegetables, promotion of regular physical activity to maintain a healthy weight, and lower sodium intake due to the reduction of processed foods. This diet has a heavy reliance on carbohydrates, although they are complex carbohydrates with a low GI. If not balanced properly, this diet can cause weight gain in some people.

Blood Type Diet

Blood Type Diet recommended by James and Peter D'Adamo recommends following a diet regimen based on person's blood type. There are 4 known blood types –A, B, AB, and O, which are strong genetic fingerprints that identify us and connect us to our ancestors. It is believed that through evolution of humankind, we changed, and our blood type evolved as well. Our body constitutions evolved and adapted to the changing environments and lifestyles throughout evolution.

Blood type O is the oldest blood type, evolved during hunting years of our ancestors, followed by type A that evolved during the agrarian time of evolution. Blood type B is next in a sequence that evolved during the movement and adaptation of human kind to a colder environment. Blood type AB is the last evolved blood type, which has a combination of characteristics of the three previous blood types. Below is a more detailed explanation and description of the characteristics of each blood type.

Blood group O — The hunter is described to be the first blood type and to have originated more than 30,000 years ago. The primary food during that time was the meat from hunted animals and some roots and plants. A high protein diet from animal sources is the recommended choice for people with this blood type. People with type O blood have a strong constitution, which contributes to their strong immune system. The personal characteristic of this blood type is a born leader, self-reliant and self-motivated. Intense physical exercises such as aerobics, running, or martial arts are well suited for people with blood group O.

Blood group A — The agrarian or cultivator dates from 20,000 years ago at the dawn of agriculture. Individuals from blood group A are recommended to eat a diet that emphasizes vegetables and is free of red meat, a diet more closely vegetarian. People with this blood type have a weaker constitution and weaker immune system and are thus more vulnerable to infections and have a sensitive digestive tract. The personal characteristics of this blood type are analytical, sensitive, and organized. It is best to engage in gentle stretching exercises for this blood type such as yoga, tai chi, and Pilates.

Blood group B— The nomad arrived 10,000 years ago. People of blood type B are the only people able to thrive on dairy products; their diet should include the most varied food groups, including meat and plants. This blood type is associated with a flexible digestive system and a strong immune system. These are flexible, creative, and balanced individuals. Moderate swimming or walking are the recommended exercise regimen for people in this group.

Blood group AB — The enigma is the most recently blood type, evolving less than 1,000 years ago. The dietary needs of this group lie between blood types A and B. This blood type has a highly tolerant immune system. The exercise regimen recommended for this group combines yoga, tai chi, and walking, hiking or cycling. The personality traits of the enigma are being charismatic, romantic, and sentimental. To get more detailed information about the Blood Type Diet and lifestyle, I would recommend reading Dr. Peter J. D'Adamo's books *Eat Right for Your Type* and *Live Right for your Type*.

What Diet Is Best For Me?

Choosing the best diet for you can be very confusing; there are so many diet books to choose from. Which one will work best? Unfortunately, there is no definite answer for each individual, and there is no one, special diet that is best for everyone either.

Dr. Roger Williams, world-renowned biochemist, published a book in 1956 called *Biochemical Individuality*. In his book, he described different individual's responses to the environment based on their physiological and anatomical variations. He stated that nutritional needs of people are different based on their genetic structure and their environment.

More research has been performed since then, and the concept of biochemical individuality proposed by Dr. Williams was developed further. It was confirmed that each person digests, absorbs, eliminates, and utilizes food differently. This means your individual requirements for calories, nutrients, vitamins, and minerals are different from everybody else's.

Only you should decide which nutritional plan is best for you. It is in your hands to review the different diets available, choose one, and experiment with it to see if it works for you. I have seen some people choose a particular diet and follow it 100%. If you prefer to diet this way, that's perfectly fine. If you can't, that's fine too. Joshua Rosenthal in his book, *Integrative Nutrition*, offers Joshua's 90–10 diet, which states you can follow your chosen diet for 90% of the time and eat foods that you crave and enjoy 10% of the time.

These numbers are just suggestions. You could try 80–20, 75–25, or a 50–50 diet at the beginning when you start eating healthy foods, and then gradually progress to eliminate as many unhealthy choices as possible. Remember, healthy eating is not a goal; it is a lifetime journey. Your body might need time to adjust to changes. When choosing the right diet, you should pay attention to several things. Is the diet balanced; does it include sufficient amounts of all 6 major components that we discussed previously: carbohydrates, proteins, healthy fats, minerals, vitamins, and fluids? Many popular diets are focused on weight loss, which they achieve by restricting calories and omitting certain foods or food groups.

Omitting food groups for a short time might help to lose weight, but unfortunately, if followed for longer periods of time, this diet might cause an imbalance and have long-term effects on your health. Make sure that the diet you choose includes sources of food that are high in fiber and antioxidants. You can also modify your chosen diet by adding any lacking nutrients with supplements of vitamins and minerals. And last but not least, choose the diet that tastes good to you and offers you choices that you will enjoy. Trust your intuition; it is your health, so the choice is yours.

Chapter 7

THE HEALING POWER OF SLEEP

"Sleep is that golden chain that ties health and our bodies together."
Thomas Dekker

We all know that sleep is important for effective body function and overall well-being. Various exercise programs and diet regimens may be used to improve health, energy, and strength; however, without sufficient sleep, these efforts might not be as successful as they could be. Lack of sleep and rest interferes with the energy necessary for exercise to be effective. Adequate sleep is more than just refreshing; it actually helps to prevent and manage diseases such as diabetes and heart disease. When we are very young, hours spent sleeping help the body grow and develop. As we get older, during the hours we sleep, the body actually repairs. During waking hours, after adequate sleep, we have boosted energy levels as well as improved concentration and memory. Additionally, sleep helps restore the body's energy, repair muscle tissue, and it also triggers the release of hormones that effect growth and appetite.

Let's take a look at what exactly regulates the sleeping pattern in our body and why we have to sleep at night. Our sleep/wake pattern is controlled by a circadian rhythm or "body clock," which is a 24-hour cycle that regulates hormone production and our sleep and wake times. The internal body clock is influenced by hormones that our body produces as well as by environmental factors such as temperature and sunlight. During the dark evening/night hours, the body produces melatonin, which helps us to fall asleep. Cortisol is another hormone that is regulated by the body clock. Cortisol, as previously discussed, is secreted by the adrenal gland and is responsible for many functions in our body. Blood levels of cortisol are highest upon waking, during the morning hours between 7:00 a.m.–8:00 a.m. Then the level slowly decreases throughout the day, with the lowest level reached at midnight. Cortisol is responsible for your feeling of hunger in the morning, for providing you with energy throughout the day, and for letting you sleep in the evening as it slowly decreases. If you happen to have abnormal adrenal function, your cortisol production is dysfunctional as well. Abnormal cortisol function could affect your sleep and wake cycle. If you are not able to get enough sleep at night, there won't be enough cortisol produced in the morning so you will have difficulty waking up. You would feel tired, have no appetite, and lack energy to function.

On the other hand, if there is too much cortisol produced during the evening or at bedtime, the result is difficulty falling asleep. Eating habits may also affect cortisol production. As was discussed previously, cortisol is responsible for glucose maintenance in the body. Adrenal fatigue negatively affects this process. When blood sugar levels drop during the night while you are sleeping, the adrenal glands increase production of cortisol, which regulate levels of blood sugar. When adrenal glands malfunction—as when they are in a state of fatigue or exhaustion—adrenalin is secreted along with the cortisol. Adrenalin produces a profound effect on the body such as a rapid heartbeat, acute alertness, and other body changes triggered by the fight or flight response. Another common complaint is "maintenance insomnia." People who experience this have no difficulty falling asleep, but they have difficulty staying asleep. They wake up during the night agitated and tense and have difficulty falling back to asleep. To avoid these nighttime waking episodes for people with adrenal fatigue, practitioners recommend a small snack consisting of protein and a complex carbohydrate at bedtime to help to keep the blood glucose at a steady level.

The circadian rhythm also controls the release of melatonin, which is the hormone responsible for inducing sleep. The rhythm is divided into 4 stages. Stages 1 and 2 are characterized by light sleep during which time one may be easily awakened. Stages 3 and 4 are deeper sleep stages, and both are very important for healing and restoring the body. It is during these stages that the pituitary gland produces the growth hormone, which is responsible for repairing body tissues. The growth hormone helps the muscles and bones absorb minerals. It also helps to remove dead cells from your tissues, and it improves immune function. Insufficient amounts of sleep on a daily basis may have a profound negative effect on your body.

Reduced sleep often causes a rise in cortisol and promotes insulin resistance. Sleep deprivation also decreases production of TSH—thyroid stimulating hormone, and may cause decreased production of the growth hormone. This could cause a premature aging of the body and other chronic conditions such as heart disease and diabetes. Studies also show that lack of adequate sleep is considered a primary cause of chronic fatigue syndrome and fibromyalgia.

How Much Sleep Do I Need?

Different people require different amounts of sleep. We all need to experience adequate time in each stage of sleep so that the brain and body get a chance to benefit. So, while it is difficult to clearly define "normal sleep," we can certainly observe that healthy individuals sleep for an average of 7–9 hours a night. The sleep rhythm also depends on age, environment, lifestyle, and diet. Each one of us is unique. Learning how to listen to your body is a key factor in discovering what works best for you. If you are not sure, you might try this simple exercise on the weekend or when on vacation: Go to sleep at your regular time at night, and record the time when you wake up naturally—without the aid of an alarm clock or anyone assisting you. Most of the time, your body will let you know when you have had enough sleep. If the sleep was satisfactory, you will awaken with energy and be generally in a positive mood. Please note that while fighting infections or during menstruation, the sleep/wake cycle is often thrown off; therefore, the best time to try to learn about your body's natural rhythm is during a time when you are relaxed and feeling well.

During the above noted experiment, please avoid taking any pills or special teas designed to assist with sleep. You might need to perform this test several times to see if your results are the same or if they differ due to environmental factors. If your results vary, take an average score and aim for the middle number of hours as your "sleep time goal." For example, if over the course of several nights you discover that there were a few nights when you slept 6 or 7 hours and a few nights that you slept 8 or 9 hours, you might aim for 7–8 hours as your sleep time goal. Keep in mind that during illness and just before and during your period, your body might need additional sleep.

Good Sleep Hygiene

There are tips for getting a good night's sleep. For instance, a bedtime routine could help you to develop healthy, regular sleeping habits. Established, predictable activities before bedtime can assist you in creating ease of sleep. Moreover, they create favorable conditions for sleeping. For effective sleep, it is vital for you to avoid certain habits. For instance, it is normally recommended that one who wishes to facilitate a good night's sleep avoid alcohol, which, based on the amount consumed, may function as a stimulant or a depressant. Examples of classic stimulants to avoid are caffeine and nicotine. You can use several methods to wind down before bedtime. These may include a warm bath, relaxation exercises, or avoiding naps during the day. You can optimize your sleep environment by making it comfortable, not too hot, noisy, cold, or bright.

Blocking out noise may help you get a better night's sleep. If you happen to be disturbed by a partner who snores, you might benefit from a pair of earplugs. Another point to consider involves light. Viewing computer or television screens before sleep may interfere with melatonin production, interfering with your sleep pattern. Therefore, you might consider getting into the habit of not using electronics before bedtime. Flickering light from computers, TV, cell phones, reading tablets, and other electronics are known to stimulate your brain and keep it awake. Set a time for yourself to wind down, and do not use these devices at least an hour before bedtime. Try to resolve emotional issues, arguments, or any emotionally stressful tasks before walking into the bedroom for the evening. Also avoid bringing work issues and work related materials to your bedroom. Beds should be used for sex and sleep. If you can't fall asleep because your mind is busy trying to solve a particular problem, get out of bed and get a piece of paper. Write out the problem you are trying to find a solution to, and analyze it. Take a few minutes to list possible solutions to the problem, choose the one that seems to work best, and come up with a plan of action. There is an excellent quote by John Steinbeck: *"It is common experience that a problem difficult at night is resolved in the morning after the committee of sleep has worked on it."* So if you can't figure out which solution to choose, promise yourself you will look at the problem again first thing in the morning, fold the paper, and go back to sleep. Most of the time, it works great for me, and when I revisit my problems in the morning, I am ready to solve them.

I Can't Fall Asleep – Help!

Insomnia is associated with difficulties in sleeping; the signs vary from one person to another. Causes of insomnia may differ but usually involve worry, stress, underlying physical conditions, menopause, drug abuse, obstructive sleep apnea, certain medications, hormonal imbalances, and restless legs syndrome. There are many treatments available for insomnia, including over-the-counter medications and natural remedies.

Several natural sleep remedies are available to address sleep problems. Relaxation exercises are an example of a natural remedy. They work by helping muscles to relax before bedtime. Note that strenuous or extensive exercises are not encouraged before bedtime. Individuals with insomnia are also advised to avoid daytime naps and encouraged to create a routine or fixed time for going to bed and waking up. Research suggests we cannot "catch up" on missed sleep, so it is not recommended that you plan on "sleeping in" to recover hours of sleep lost the night before. Herbal remedies are often used as alternative treatments for sleep challenges. The most commonly used are L-theanine, wild lettuce, valerian, passionflower, and Jamaican dogwood. Other remedies include melatonin, lemon balm and 5-HTP (5-Hydroxy-L-Tryptophan). Please consult with your health care practitioner to find out which of the natural remedies is safe for you. Since insomnia may be an indicator of more serious health issues, you should consult your health care practitioner about sleep patterns and discuss recommended treatments. In many cases, once underlying medical conditions (i.e. hormonal imbalances) are resolved, insomnia resolves as well.

Chapter 8

THE HEALING POWER OF MOVEMENT

"Those who think they have no time for exercise will sooner or later have to find time for illness." Edward Stanley

Getting the appropriate amount of and kind of exercise benefits nearly all aspects of your life and health. Physical activity is vital in order to enhance youthful agility throughout the years. An added benefit of keeping the body active is that it may help to prevent certain degenerative diseases. Exercise can help with weight control, often improves mood, builds strong bones and muscles, and may increase your longevity.

Regular physical activity is one of the best lifestyle changes that you can make to ensure a healthy, long, and active life. It can reduce your risk of developing diabetes, cardiovascular disease, and high blood pressure and can also enhance glycemic control and insulin sensitivity. Regular exercise may help you to sleep better, strengthen your immune system, reduce menstrual discomfort, and yes, might even improve the quality of your sex life. I hope you are convinced by now; so let's get started.

What Exercises Do I Need?

An unfortunate side effect of progress in technology is that our physical activity levels declined, which negatively affected our physical health. Statistics show that the average American adult walks less than a mile a day. Common questions often asked include, "How much exercise is needed?" "What types of exercises are best and when is the best time to exercise?" According to the American Heart Association, adults 18 years of age and older need to do at least 2 hours of an activity of moderate intensity each week and muscle strengthening exercises twice a week. Exercises such as brisk walking, playing tennis, bike riding, and gardening are considered moderate intensity exercises. Jogging, swimming, jumping rope, running, hiking, or group activities such as Zumba or step aerobics are considered vigorous intensity activities. Muscle-strengthening activities you might consider including in your routine twice a week may include yoga, lifting weights, resistance band exercises, and body-weight resistance activities like push-ups and sit-ups.

All these activities sound great; however, common complaints that I hear from busy women include not having enough time to go to the gym 3 times a week or that they get more tired than invigorated after exercising—which reduces rather than increases energy. I also see women who have tried to start an exercise regimen but unfortunately hurt themselves because their body was so out of shape. Well let's see if we can find answers to all these questions and situations.

What Exercises Work For Me?

In answer to the question about the type of exercise to choose, an individualized approach is required. As previously mentioned, we each have a different body constitution, muscle strength, individual potential, and a starting condition. These all need to be considered when choosing an exercise regimen. You should choose appropriate physical activities to avoid injuries while exercising. Dr. Arkady Lipnitsky, Chiropractor, Diplomat of the American Chiropractic Rehabilitation Board, and Director of Chiropractic and Rehabilitation at Pain Physicians New York, advises that generally, healthy individuals can engage in any form of exercise. However, people with certain medical conditions should choose appropriate physical activities based on experts' recommendations to avoid injuries.

Strenuous exercise may create small microscopic tears in muscle tissue, joint pain, torn muscles, as well as bone fractures. Therefore, training slowly and consistently to avoid injury during exercise is important. Dr. Lipnitsky says that in his practice, he treats a wide variety of patients for exercise related injuries. Some of his patients are professional athletes, musicians, and dancers, who injure themselves from overusing their muscles and joints. Some patients are people who injured themselves after having chosen an inappropriate exercise regimen; specifically, after having not exercised for a long time, they chose exercises that were too strenuous for their current physical condition. For beginners, Dr. Lipnitsky recommends that you consult an exercise specialist or a personal trainer to assess your body strengths and weaknesses and help you develop an exercise regimen that is safe and individualized for you.

What Should Be Included In My Exercise Regimen?

There are several components to an appropriate physical exercise regimen, says Marcin Machula, Performance Enhancement Specialist (PES) certified by the National Academy of Sports Medicine. First, it is most important to assess your body's condition, your posture, movement, and your exercise performance. The fitness assessment builds the foundation for the entire exercise program. It helps to make an appropriate selection of flexibility, cardiovascular, core, balance, and strengthening exercises. From the gathered information, more individualized training programs can be built for your specific goals and needs.

Secondly, if you are new to fitness activities, it's very beneficial to focus on exercises that engage the whole body, for instance push-ups, squats, standing cable rows, single leg shoulder scaptions, or Swiss ball bridges. Improving muscular endurance, stability, and coordination are very important training components at the beginner level of training. Building a solid foundation is paramount.

Thirdly, core training has become a popular fitness trend in recent years and a common method of training used by personal trainers. The objective of core training is to help you to strengthen the deep and superficial muscles that stabilize, align, and move the trunk of the body, especially the abdominals and muscles of the back. Physical therapists prescribe core exercises for patients with low back problems, and more recently, core training has become popular among athletes to help improve sports performance. A week core is a fundamental problem inherent to inefficient movement that may lead to predictable patterns of injury. A proper core training program could help you gain neuromuscular control, stability, muscular endurance, strength, and power of the core.

Finally, cardiovascular exercises, such as jogging, swimming, cycling, skipping and weight lifting, will help to enhance your cardiovascular health. Such exercises should become your routine and optimum for maximum benefits.

How Do I Choose A Physical Activity?

Before you do anything, I would advise you to see your health care practitioner to get a checkup and discuss your exercise plans to find out if you have any restrictions to exercising. The next step—especially if you are out of shape and have not been exercising for some time—is to find yourself an exercise specialist. Most gyms now offer a session with an exercise specialist or a personal trainer when you sign up for a membership. Discuss with your personal trainer what will work best for you, and try to choose an activity that is safe and beneficial for your needs and that you will enjoy doing. Below is the list of suggested exercise routines:

Power walking is an aerobic workout that involves speed blasts and slow recovery breaks to offer adequate intensity for improving cardio-respiratory fitness. Although power walking is effective for burning calories quickly and enhancing muscle strength, it is associated with certain muscle injuries particularly when done poorly through exaggerated strides. Build up your walking routine slowly, adding distance and speed as you progress from day to day. Power walking is the easiest and the least expensive exercise since a pair of good supportive running shoes is all that is required.

Jogging or running involves maintaining a particular stride at a restrained speed for a given distance outside or on a treadmill. As an aerobic exercise, jogging is a fundamental means of burning more calories, improving heart health, and increasing bone density. Jogging, however, is not for everyone. It may cause knee injuries and chronic pain, so start gradually and build up slowly as tolerated.

Weight training, such as biceps curls, pull-down, lunges, and squats, involves the lifting of weight to build muscles. It is an effective method of improving bone density, enhancing the rate of metabolism, and reducing muscle shrinkage during aging. Weight training also leads to strong muscles and stability. Weight training, however, is associated with stress of the musculoskeletal system, which might lead to tiny microscopic tears in the affected muscle tissue. Start with light weights first as you incorporate weight training 2–3 times per week, and then gradually build up to heavier weights and greater intensity of exercise. Busy moms of small babies and toddlers might skip this type of exercise since they do plenty of weight lifting by carrying their babies. For those who carry infants and toddlers, it's important to remember to use proper body mechanics including avoiding bending down at the waist when lifting as this may injure your back. Instead, practice squatting at the knees while keeping your back as straight as possible, and then use your leg muscles to elevate your body with the infant or toddler close to your torso.

HIIT—High Intensity Interval Training is based on "short yet intense exercises and then short rest or recovery time." HIIT exercises, such as cardio workouts, drills, and brisk walks, improve oxygen consumption and metabolic activities. These results facilitate fat loss for nearly a day after the exercise. HIIT may not be suitable for individuals who cannot endure intense training. This form of exercise is perfect for people who are already fit and have been exercising regularly but who want to add a short and quality workout to their busy schedules.

Here are some popular HIIT training exercises:
- Insanity
- FOCUS T25 workout
- PiYo workout
- 7-Minute Workout
- P90X

These types of exercise programs are designed for different levels of fitness, offer a variety of exercises that are fun to do, and are generally short in duration. If you are interested, try them out and see which one works best for you.

Yoga consists of exercise elements that entail different body postures —mainly stretching and strengthening of the musculature—and is geared to bring balance to the mental, emotional, and spiritual aspects of your life. Different types of yoga exist, and your individual preference will help you decide what best suits you. Here are the most popular types of yoga:

Bikram Yoga—also referred to as "hot yoga"— is performed at 95–105 degree temperatures. This type of yoga focuses on muscular endurance and strength, cardiovascular flexibility, detoxification, and weight loss. You will need to remember to drink plenty of fluids before, during, and after the session to prevent dehydration.

Hatha—is a basic form of yoga that is easy to learn and incorporates the basic principles of all yoga styles, such as Asanas (postures), Pranayama (regulated breathing), and meditation (Dharana & Dhyana). It is considered one of the easiest types for beginners.

Kripalu—is a gentle form of yoga referred to as the yoga of consciousness. It allows you to hold poses designed to help the body release spiritual and emotional blockages.

Kundalini—includes chanting, meditation, and breathing exercises designed to help awaken your energy and draw it upward.

Viniyoga—is a healing and gentle yoga tailored to the individual. It is used as a therapeutic exercise for people with injuries.

Do your research and find a beginners' class in your area. Consult your instructor on do's and don'ts for beginners so you can avoid injury to your muscles and joints. If you don't have access to your chosen yoga class, there are great yoga books and DVDs available for your use. Just make sure you start with a beginners' video or book.

Exercise Opportunities During the Day

If you have absolutely no time to go to a gym or to sign up for a class, that is okay. You might be getting more exercise than you realize. If this is the case, all you need to do is make what you are already doing work better for you. Assessing your daily routine will help you realize there are many ways in which you are likely already very active and ways to sneak additional exercise into your lifestyle.

Remember that everything you do throughout the day that makes you move counts as exercise. This might include walking your dog, taking your kids to school, working in the garden, cleaning your house, and even doing laundry. To receive the most benefit from the physical activity you are already doing in the form of household chores, you will need to concentrate on your body as it is moving to ensure proper posture and body mechanics. You can add speed, hold a position a moment longer, or add a stretch or two between activities.

Adding steps to your daily routine may be easier than you think. For instance, when shopping, you can park your car a few spaces farther from the market or store, or if you have more time, you can park your car a couple of blocks away from your destination and walk at brisk pace the rest of the way. Burn your calories not electricity by taking stairs rather than elevators. Pace around the house or climb steps while you talk on the phone.

Get up and walk, do push-ups or sit-ups during TV commercials, or stretch your calves and rotate your ankles while sitting at your desk or computer. Don't forget that playing with your kids is also a form of exercise. Take your kids outside to play a game of tag instead of watching TV together as a way to share quality time while being physically active. This helps them form healthy lifestyle habits as well.

Every minute of your daily activity counts. That means if one day you walk your kids to school in the morning for 10 minutes, climb stairs at work for 5 minutes, do active household chores for 20 minutes, and play with your kids for another 25 minutes, that is already a whole hour of physical activity that day. Last, but not least, is my personal favorite: **Sexercise**—yes, sexual activity is also a form of exercise as it helps burn anywhere between 100–300 calories per session.

Home Gym or Fitness Club?

Getting physically fit doesn't have to be complicated. If you decide to sign up for a membership in a local gym or a fitness club, that's great. Be sure to ask if the facility offers a session with an exercise specialist or a personal trainer. If they don't, ask them to recommend one. If going to the gym is not an option, you could invest in a home gym. It is cheaper, more convenient, and can be accessed by you and your family any hour of the day and in any weather. You can use a home gym whenever you have a few free minutes, ideally for 5–20 minute intervals. To establish a home gym, you don't have to purchase any fancy or expensive equipment. All you might need is a yoga mat, a bench, some weights and a comfortable place to store them. Other equipment to consider is a Swiss/stability ball, dumbbells in varieties of weights, resistance bands, and foam rollers. If you decide to invest in equipment that is more expensive, buying a portable stepping machine or cycling bike for cardio workouts is a great choice. They don't take up a lot of space and can be used at any time for a short period. In Part 4 of this book, Marcin Machula, PES, provides a beginner-level exercise regimen of simple-to-do exercises, which can be performed at work or at home with intervals throughout the day.

Chapter 9

BEAUTIFUL YOU

"Beauty is how you feel inside and it reflects in your eyes." Sophie Loren

Growing up, we probably all had favorite images of beautiful princesses and wanted to grow up to be as beautiful as them. When younger, we probably couldn't define exactly what beauty was, and as grownups, some of us are still not able to define exactly what beauty is. Beauty is such a general concept and can be defined and expressed in so many ways.

Beauty is defined and shaped by our beliefs, values, culture, society, and everything else that affects our life. Kahlil Gibran has an excellent quote: *"Beauty is not in the face; beauty is a light in the heart."* I truly believe that beauty radiates from within a woman. It is the way she smiles, listens to her inner self and others, radiates positive energy toward others, laughs, and enjoys her own life while bringing joy to the lives of people around her. A beautiful woman is one who knows her life purpose and lives her life to the fullest, enjoying every moment of it.

While it is absolutely fabulous to be glowing and radiating beauty from the inside, in this chapter, I would like to discuss how to compliment your inner beauty and be beautiful from the outside as well. It is important to follow basic everyday hygiene and keep yourself clean, but it is also important for every woman to pay attention to her appearance. Feel good about yourself and your looks; get a regular haircut and color if needed; do your nails; buy yourself some new and nice clothes and shoes, and make yourself feel happy when you look in the mirror.

Beautiful Hair

Historically, women's hair was viewed as one of the attributes of femininity. Today, a woman's hair goes beyond her femininity and is often a reflection of her identity, her self-esteem, her freedom, her beauty, her thoughts and beliefs, and her ways of expressing herself. Let's take a look what you need to do to have beautiful hair.

First, it is important to find a knowledgeable hairstylist who will help you to choose a hairstyle and color, if needed, that will compliment you and your complexion. Regardless of the hair color and hairstyle you choose, there are simple basic hair-care tips every woman should know and follow to have beautiful and silky tresses.

Our diet and lifestyle play a significant role in how our hair feels and looks. It is important to make sure to consume foods that are high in minerals and vitamins, such as selenium, vitamins A, E, and omega-3 fatty acids. Sometimes, problems with hair may be a result of underlying hormonal imbalances, which we discussed previously. In many cases, once hormonal levels are restored, skin and hair texture improves automatically. Sometimes it can be a stressful lifestyle or life changing events such as pregnancy, surgery, or other chronic medical conditions that cause a woman to lose her hair. Regardless of the reason, it is important to always address underlying problems and follow the simple hair-care strategies listed below:

Keep your hair clean. Our hair is very absorbent, and it attracts and holds molecules of polluted substances from the air. We are talking about the smell of smoke and dangerous chemicals in our environment. Did you ever had the experience of spending hours in the kitchen cooking and later couldn't shake the smell of the food from your hair? Washing your hair helps to remove the chemicals that you might have absorbed from the air and to prevent them being absorbed into your system.

Choose your hair color and style to compliment your face shape and complexion. Your hair color and style might make you look younger or older, thinner or heavier, might compliment your skin complexion, or make you look pale and haggard. So choose your hair color and style carefully. If you are not sure, you can experiment with online tools such as thehairstyler.com where you can upload your picture and try different hair colors and styles. Or you can visit a store and tryout different wigs and see which ones look best on you. You can also ask for suggestions from your hairstylist, who might recommend a hairstyle and color that will suit you and your hair texture the best.

Trim, color, and style your hair regularly. Choose your hairstyle by taking into consideration how busy your schedule is and if you are able to style your hair at home. Shorter hairstyles need more maintenance and attention, while with longer hairstyles, you have more options of either letting it lie naturally, putting it in a ponytail, or using hair accessories. Keep your hair clean and neat to prevent it from looking unkempt and frazzled.

Treat your hair gently. Avoid over-processing and overheating your hair. Chemicals in hair coloring and high heat settings on your flat or curling iron can damage your hair, causing changes in your hair texture and hair loss. Choose natural and organic hair coloring products with fewer chemicals in them. Give color holidays to your hair by changing your hairstyle and color back to your natural looks, and don't color your hair for several months. Treat your hair with nourishing and soothing creams or oil treatments to revitalize and to support your hair.

Change your hairstyle and color occasionally to give yourself a new look. It doesn't have to be something drastic as coloring your hair blue or purple (even though you might try this. I have seen some amazing hairstyles with these colors). Keeping the same hairstyle might look like you are stuck in the past and out of touch with the times. It is not uncommon for women who get married and stop dating to keep the same hairstyle for next 10, 15 or 20 years, if not more. Probably, these women are used to their hairstyle, feel comfortable with it, and don't have time to choose a new one. I will encourage you to try a new look and see how positively it will affect your self-esteem and your mood. You will feel more sensual and sexual, and I am sure it will not go unnoticed by your partner.

Protect your hair from damage caused by direct sun exposure. Sun exposure can cause damage to protein in your hair called keratin, which will make your hair thinner and more breakable. Choose hair-care products that are free of chemicals and contain sunscreen.

Selecting appropriate hair-care products and following an appropriate hair-care routine might also have a significant effect on your hair texture. Depending on your hair type— oily, normal, or dry—how often you wash your hair, and what type of shampoo you use, your routine will be different. Our hair needs lubrication as does any other part of our body, so if you have dry hair, choose a shampoo appropriate for your hair type, which will provide needed moisture and lubrication to your hair. Also, you might consider washing your hair every other day instead of daily to preserve its moisture. Coloring and bleaching your hair tends to cause damage to your hair structure, causing it to dry more. Ask your hairstylist to recommend a hair product for you that will support and nourish your processed hair. For those with oily hair, find a hair-care shampoo that will help you to balance the pH level of your scalp and your hair oil production. Using fewer hair styling products, such as mousses, gels, and hairspray, will keep your hair less oily longer. Depending on how fast your hair gets oily, you might need to wash it once or twice a day. Choose organic and chemical free shampoos and hair-care products.

I AM LOSING MY HAIR—HELP!

Hair loss has always been considered a male problem; however, statistics show that women are also likely to lose their hair as they age. The majority of women who lose their hair notice it in their 50s, but it might happen at any age and is affected by different reasons. According to the American Academy of Dermatology, it is normal for women to lose approximately 50–100 strands of hair each day. These old shedding hairs are usually replaced with the new ones. If you notice that your hairbrush and your shower has more shed hair than it used to, you might need to investigate what is causing you to loose hair. The causes of hair loss are different, and the most common ones are listed below:

- Unbalanced diet
- Physical or emotional stress
- Menopause
- Hormonal imbalances
- Hereditary
- Absence of proper hair care
- Autoimmune disorders

What Treatment Options Are Available?

To find a solution for hair loss, we need to find a reason why it is happening to begin with. A person suffering hair loss needs to be tested for hormonal imbalances and nutritional deficiencies since these two issues seem to be the most common causes of hair loss. A variety of treatment options for hair loss are available today, including Rogaine, estrogen and progesterone containing contraceptives, and platelet rich plasma therapy (PRP).

Minoxidil (Rogaine)

Minoxidil was originally used as a type of blood pressure lowering medication (antihypertensive). Patients that were taking this medication noticed a common side effect of excessive hair growth (hypertrichosis). Later, researchers found out that applying Minoxidil directly to the scalp has a similar effect and can also stimulate hair growth.

Minoxidil doesn't grow new hair. You need to have live and active hair follicles for Minoxidil to work by prolonging the growth phase of the hair shaft. Today, we have a variety of hair-care products such as Rogaine on the market that are used to treat hair loss. Most of these products are applied topically to the scalp for extended periods of time and improve hair growth by improving blood circulation to the scalp. Results are usually seen in 3–4 months.

Minoxidil containing products are usually well tolerated and are available over the counter in your local pharmacy. Common side effects include burning scalp, facial hair growth, inflammation or soreness at the root of the hair, and reddened skin. Minoxidil could also cause rare side effects such as vasodilation, flushing, and hypotension. Contact your health care provider to see if Minoxidil is safe for you.

Estrogen and Progesterone

Estrogen and progesterone pills and creams, such as Diane-35 and Diane-50, may be an effective treatment for women who are losing their hair due to hormonal imbalances such as menopause or whose estrogen or progesterone are imbalanced for other reasons. Cyproterone acetate with ethinylestradiol is sold under the brand names Diane-35 and Diane-50. These contraceptive tablets are prescribed in Europe for women with hormonal alopecia. Currently, both versions of this contraceptive are not available in the US. However, your health care provider might help you to identify your underlying hormonal imbalance, and in many cases, treating the hormonal imbalance will reverse your hair loss as well.

Platelet Rich Plasma Therapy (PRP)

PRP is a relatively new treatment used for men and women with hair loss. PRP is an invasive, nonsurgical therapeutic option available to people with hair loss. The PRP is performed by a certified medical professional in a clinical setting where a blood sample from your body is obtained and prepared by spinning it in a special machine. The specimen obtained is a liquid with the highly concentrated platelet rich plasma, which contains many growths factors. Your scalp is prepared with a special micro needling device, and the platelet rich liquid is injected into your scalp under local anesthesia. The growth factors contained in a PRP will help to stimulate hair follicle growth.

This procedure needs to be performed every three to four months to be effective, and PRP treatments can help create new blood vessels in your scalp and stimulate hair growth. PRP is considered relatively safe and does not cause allergic or hypersensitive reactions. After the treatment, you might experience a mild inflammatory response at the procedure site, which might cause tenderness of your scalp for several days.

PRP is effective for people with live hair follicles. If your hair follicles are damaged or lost, this procedure is not for you. PRP is also contraindicated for people with a history of diabetes, blood-clotting disorder, active infection of the scalp, a history of shingles, or those taking immunosuppressant and blood-thinning medications.

Unwelcome Body Hair

Now, let's discuss body hair, something we all have, some of us more some less. How we deal with it depends a lot on our personal values and how we feel about this issue. For some women, having smooth skin, regardless of whether in places visible or not, just makes them feel better and more sensual. However, having extra body hair might be more than something that is just unpleasant to look at. There is also a medical condition called hirsutism—a condition of unwanted, male-pattern hair growth in women. Hirsutism results in excessive amounts of stiff and pigmented hair on body areas where men typically grow hair — face, chest, back, and legs. As discussed previously, this condition could be directly related to a hormonal imbalance such as polycystic ovary syndrome (PCOS), hyperthyroidism, and adrenal dysfunction. The primary treatment for hirsutism should be diagnosing and regulating the underlying hormonal imbalances. Aesthetic treatment options for unwanted hair are the old standard shaving and waxing and new modalities of different intense pulsed light (IPL), electrolysis, and laser treatments.

Types of Lasers Used For Hair Removal

Laser is an acronym for *Light Amplification by Stimulated Emission of Radiation.* Laser hair removal is a treatment that uses lasers to target the roots of hair underneath the skin's surface. No single laser is ideal for every individual. Depending on your skin and hair color, some lasers will be more effective than others. There are a variety of lasers on the market, some more effective than others on different skin tones, hair colors, and treatment areas. Laser hair removal can also be performed on any part of the body. A series of treatments are usually needed for hair removal to be permanent. How do you choose the best laser for you? Let's take a look at the different laser treatments available.

The Ruby Laser works by the beam of the laser being absorbed by the melanin pigment in the hair and is not effective for use on lighter, white/gray hair. Is safe to be used on patients with a fair skin complexion but might cause burns on dark and tanned skin.

The Alexandrite Laser is the fastest hair removal laser. It penetrates deep into the layers of the skin. It is suitable for patients with fair to olive complexions and might cause pigment changes such as darkening or lightening of the skin.

The Diode Laser has a longer wavelength than the ruby and alexandrite lasers, which allows deep penetration into the skin. It is safe for dark skinned people but not effective for use on lighter and finer hair.

The Nd: YAG laser can be used on all skin types, including tanned and dark skin. It provides a less effective treatment for white and light hair.

Intense pulsed light (IPL) is used for hair removal, but its primary use is to treat skin pigmentation problems. IPL works best on patients with dark hair and fair skin.

How to Choose the Right Laser Treatment

Laser hair removal has become a very popular treatment option in recent years. Laser hair removal is considered an effective and safe procedure if done by an educated and certified provider, says Svetlana Kotlovskiy, a Certified Laser Specialist and Director of Green Planet Spa in New York. If not performed correctly, there can be some side effects to laser hair removal, such as skin damage. Svetlana Kotlovskiy suggests that women follow these guidelines to choose a laser hair-removal treatment:

• Ask who will perform the procedure and if that person has proper certifications for laser treatment.

- Schedule a consultation and discuss which laser type would be best for your skin, and ask for a spot test to see how your body will react to the treatment.

- Ask how many treatments you will need and how often you should schedule your sessions. The number and frequency of treatments will be different depending on your hair type and the body part being treated. Laser hair removal works best when a hair follicle is targeted during a special phase of growth—anagen phase—which might be different for each body part. For instance, most of the body hair above the waistline has approximately a 4–6 week cycle, while hair below the waist has 6–8 weeks cycle. This means you should be scheduling your sessions for upper body parts every 4–6 weeks and lower body parts every 6–8 weeks. The timing might vary in each individual, but these are the average recommendations.

- Check the cleaning procedures of the clinic and the standards they use to clean their equipment. Since most places use the same machine for hair removal on different body parts, it is important that the machine is being cleaned properly with hospital/medical grade wipes or cleaning solution after each use.

- There are certain contraindications for laser hair removal that you should be aware of, you need to make sure you notify your technician if you have them. This procedure is contraindicated if you are taking medications that cause photosensitivity, such as certain antibiotics, have a medical condition causing you to be more photosensitive, viral or bacterial infections, or are pregnant.

- Laser hair removal is an ongoing process and might require 4–8 session to be successful, so be patient. You will need to shave the area before the procedure. After the treatment, your hair will fall out in 1–2 weeks. After each treatment, your hair will grow slower and thinner with a 20 to 40% reduction in amount.

LOVE THE SKIN YOU ARE IN

Our skin is our biggest body organ, which covers us from head to toe and can tell us a lot about our health and our age. Healthy skin has elasticity, turgor, is glowing and radiant. Multiple products on the market today can help you to disguise your wrinkles and spots and help you to get that dewy and glowing skin. However, these are only temporary solutions, and once you take off that makeup, you are left with lifeless skin with whatever wrinkles and blemishes it has. Proper daily skin care can help you keep your skin looking and feeling younger and healthier for many years.

Daily Skin Regimen

A daily skin-care regimen is very important and doesn't have to be complicated and expensive. Expensive laser treatments and injectable rejuvenating procedures are very popular today, which is great, and they do have their place in helping us recapture our youth (I will discuss them later in the chapter). However, many women spend a lot of time and money for these procedures while neglecting a simple daily skin-care regimen. Proper skin care can help your skin to feel and look younger and, to a certain extent, prevent the aging of your skin. Ellen Gavrielov, a certified specialist in cosmeceuticals and fragrance production and marketing, says that before you go into more details about skin care, you will need to know what your skin type is in order to carry out an effective skin-care regimen. She states that our skin type is determined by our genetics and ethnicity. It can be directly measured by the size of the sebaceous glands and by the amount of oil produced in the skin, especially in the T-zone area. Natural oil secretions from the sebaceous glands help protect our skin from environmental damage and aging. The T-zone is the center area of the face corresponding to the forehead, nose,

155

and chin (shaped as a letter T) and has more oil glands and larger pores than the other parts of the face. There are 5 skin types, which we will discuss in detail: normal, dry, combination, oily, and sensitive.

Skin Types

Normal: This skin type displays a smooth texture with no evidence of dryness or excessive oiliness. The follicles are not enlarged, and there are no visible blemishes, greasy patches, or flaky areas. Sebum production, water moisture content, and cell renewal are well balanced. Normal skin has a natural resilience that helps to prevent common problems such as broken capillaries, spots, or redness. Those with normal skin types have a rosy, clear surface, and fine pores. The goal for those with this skin type is to maintain the skin health with the right skin-care regimen.

Dry: This skin type does not produce enough oil. The follicles tend to be small, which indicates that sebum production is minimal. Dry skin results in tightness and flaking. The skin appears dull, especially on the cheeks and around the eyes. It usually lacks elasticity and has fine lines and wrinkles emphasized. Dry skin types need a skin-care regimen that will stimulate oil production.

Combination: Combination skin is rather dry in some parts of the face and oily in the T-zone area. The T-zone tends to become oily as it has more sebaceous glands and larger pores. The surrounding skin or outer areas of the face, such as the cheeks and around the eyes, can be dry and sometimes appears flaky. Combination skin requires a skin-care regimen that will balance the oil and water content on the skin. Deep cleansing, regular exfoliation (which we will discuss), and the use of water-based products will help balance out the skin.

Oily: This skin type is characterized by an increased amount of oil production due to overactive sebaceous glands. Oily skin appears shiny, often with enlarged pores over most of the face, and has a waxy texture.

Oily skin is prone to blackheads and other blemishes because of the amount of oil that gets trapped or clogged in its pores. However, on the flip side, it ages at a slower rate than other skin types. The main goal for those with this skin type is to balance the oil production. The common mistake is using an aggressive approach to remove or strip oil from the skin. The excessive dryness that results causes the body to overcompensate by signaling the sebaceous glands to produce more oil to replace the lost moisture. This skin type requires proper exfoliation to eliminate the dead skin cells from clogging the pores further and the use of water-based products that will hydrate the skin without the extra oil.

Sensitive: This skin type is characterized by being more delicate than the others, with a lower amount of pigment, a thin epidermis, and blood vessels close to the skin surface, causing redness. Sensitive skin is often the result of a defect in the epidermal lipid barrier layer—which is the skin's protective outer layer—allowing irritants, bacteria, and allergens to penetrate the skin and cause adverse reactions. The visible signs of a skin reaction include redness, dermatitis, chafing, broken veins, capillaries, and mild bruising. Sensitive skin needs to be cleansed and maintained with hypoallergenic and unscented products, as many ingredients, including the synthetic chemicals in conventional skin-care treatments, are unsuitable for sensitive skin. Products formulated with natural organic ingredients are safer in this respect. The goal for those with sensitive skin is to soothe and calm the skin, which requires a high degree of protection against hostile weather conditions and ultraviolet radiation.

Ellen's Six-Step Guide to Skin-Care Regimen

Cleanse — Even if you don't wear makeup, it's very important to wash your face with a cleanser and not body or hand soap. A skin-care regimen starts with a good cleanser—but let's first talk about why you need to make sure your skin is cleaned properly, no matter what skin type you have. Facial cleansers remove makeup, pollutants, bacteria, and unwanted debris off your face. When using the right cleanser for your skin type and condition, the ingredients in the formula can help alleviate sensitivity, soften dry skin, or care for whatever your skin needs. In addition, it's important to recognize that properly cleansing the skin prepares your skin to absorb any products applied after, such as a serum or moisturizer. When you cleanse, you clear out your pores, allowing the moisturizer to penetrate into your skin for maximum effectiveness. Facial products are formulated specifically for the sebaceous glands on the skin of your face. Soaps used for hand and body cleansing are much too harsh for the face as they strip off all the oils that help protect your skin. These soaps also contain ingredients that clog the pores or can sensitize the skin. Cleansing should be done twice a day: once in the morning before applying moisturizers and makeup and the second time at night to remove the makeup or debris trapped on our skin. The best way to cleanse is to dampen the skin with water, take a pea-sized amount of your cleanser and with both hands, apply the cleanser to your skin, and lather in a circular motion covering all areas except the eyes.

Exfoliate — Exfoliation is an important step in skin treatment and should only be part of your regimen up to 4 times a week after cleansing the skin. Exfoliating removes the dead cells that build up on the surface of the skin and provides substantial improvement to dry, acne-prone, and photo-damaged skin conditions. Just as cleansing the pores helps other products penetrate deeper, exfoliating the skin helps to remove the barrier and buildup of old cells to freshen the skin, allowing further penetration of treatment serums. There are two methods of exfoliation: mechanical and chemical. Mechanical/physical exfoliants work by eliminating dead skin cells on the surface with the use of superfine abrasive agents, such as crushed cranberry seeds, oatmeal, rice bran, etc. Tools such as facial brushes or facial sponges can be used as well. Chemical exfoliants work by dissolving the "glue" that binds skin cells together. Once it is penetrated into the skin, the chemical agent dissolves the glue, allowing the dead cells to shed and additionally stimulating cell renewal. There are 4 types of chemical exfoliating agents: Alpha Hydroxy Acids, Beta Hydroxy Acids, enzymes, and retinol. Alpha Hydroxy Acids (AHA) are water soluble and therefore only exfoliate the upper layer of the skin. The most common AHAs include lactic acid, glycolic acid, and mandelic acid.

- Lactic acid is derived from milk. It hydrates the skin, increases natural barrier lipids in the outer layer of skin, and is used to lighten skin discolorations, such as hyperpigmentation.
- Glycolic acid is derived from cane sugar. Because it is made up small molecules, it penetrates the skin easily allowing a deeper exfoliation.
- Mandelic acid is extracted from bitter almonds; has larger molecules than most AHAs, making it less irritating on the skin; and has antibacterial properties, which are beneficial to acne sufferers.

Beta Hydroxy Acids (BHA) are oil soluble, which means that they not only exfoliate the upper layer of skin, but also penetrate deep into the pores to exfoliate the excess sebum and dead skin cells built up inside the pores. Although BHA penetrates deeper than AHA, BHA is less irritating due to its anti-inflammatory properties. Salicylic acid is the only form of BHA. It is an organic acid that is extracted from the bark of a willow tree. Salicylic acid is both antimicrobial and anti-inflammatory and is frequently used to treat blackheads, whiteheads, and acne.

Retinol, also known as Vitamin A, is an antioxidant and considered a cell-communicating ingredient. Unlike AHAs and BHA that exfoliate the upper layers of the skin, retinol works by stimulating the cell turnover from the deeper layers of skin. Retinol is best used in conjunction with AHAs and BHA to help shed the dead skin retinol helped to accelerate. Retinol has been shown to improve the visible signs of photo aging as well as normal aging when used on a daily basis.

Enzyme exfoliants work by digesting keratin protein and breaking down the bonds holding the dead cells on the skin. Additionally, the use of enzymes rarely cause irritation and help strengthen the skin with its natural antioxidant properties. The most commonly used enzymes are papain, bromelain and pumpkin.

- Papain is found naturally in unripe green papayas and contains high amounts of vitamin A, vitamin C, and vitamin K.
- Bromelain is found in pineapple stems. In addition to its exfoliating properties, this enzyme helps rebuild collagen and reduce redness. Bromelain contains vitamin C and has potent anti-inflammatory properties.
- Pumpkin and its seeds contain vitamin A, vitamin C, essential fatty acids, vitamin E, and zinc. The molecular structure of pumpkin is small and therefore can penetrate deeper into the skin. Pumpkin brightens and assists with healing the skin.

Tone —Toners are liquids used for cleansing or exfoliating just before applying moisturizer. Toning the skin removes the residue left behind by cleansers and helps to temporarily tighten open follicles. Additionally, toning restores the skin's natural pH after cleansing and can help certain skin conditions, depending on the type of ingredients in your toner. Spray the toner directly onto the skin, and use a cotton pad to spread it around. This method also helps you transfer the residue onto the cotton pad. Toners vary in strength as some may have higher alcohol content than others.

Treat — This step pertains to those who need to treat a variety of skin conditions such as dehydration, hyperpigmentation, acne, or sensitized skin. Serums contain the most potent dose of antioxidants, peptides, and skin brighteners. Many treatment serums are formulated with very high concentrations of active ingredients and are made of very small molecules and thus are extremely effective. Serums are used after the toning step and before the moisturizer are applied. They can be used twice a day, depending on the active ingredients. Any products containing brightening agents are recommended for use in the evening when the skin is not exposed to sunlight. However, if you choose to apply serums in the morning, be sure to protect your skin with an SPF containing product to avoid pigmentation.

Moisturize — Our skin has many important functions, including the prevention of water loss. Moisturizers help keep our skin smooth and healthy, but they also provide protection from harmful irritants in the environment and are formulated to add moisture to the skin. The ingredients used in body lotions can clog pores on facial skin. Avoid using body lotions on your face as this could cause skin irritation or breakouts. Each skin type requires a different form of moisturizing emulsion, containing higher or lower levels of oil. Oil-based emollients are denser and are best for people who have dry skin that needs intensive moisturizing. Water-based emollients, on the other hand, are lighter and less greasy, which makes them ideal for people with normal, oily, or acne-prone skin. Other ingredients that moisturizers contain include vitamins, minerals, plant extracts, and fragrances or essential oils used as fragrance.

Protect — The final stage in our daily routine is of the up most importance as it will help keep our skin healthy and youthful. Let me explain why. The sun is a source of the full spectrum of ultraviolet (UV) light, which is invisible to the human eye. The three classifications of UV light are UVA, UVB, and UVC. UVC rays are absorbed by the ozone layer and therefore do not reach the earth. UVA light is deeply absorbed by the epidermis because of its short wavelengths and is the dominant tanning ray. It accounts of up to 95% of the ultraviolet rays that reach the earth's surface. UVA light is considered to be made of aging rays as it weakens the skin's collagen and elastin fibers, resulting in skin tissues that sag and wrinkle. Prolonged ultraviolet light exposure not only leads to hyperpigmentation, free radical damage, elastin deterioration, and capillary damage, but might also leads to skin cancer.

UVB rays are longer wavelengths that are responsible for skin reddening and sunburn due to the ray's penetration into the dermis. UVB light affects melanocytes, the cells of the epidermis that are responsible for producing melanin. Melanin is responsible for the protection of our skin and for the pigment that gives human skin, hair, and eyes their color. Although UVB rays account for only 5% of the sunlight that reaches the earth's surface, these rays are equally damaging to the skin and eyes. UVB rays play a significant role in the development of skin cancer and an influential role in tanning and photo aging. It is crucial to take the necessary precautions when exposed to sunlight. The final step in your skin-care regimen is the application of a sunscreen to your face and body.

SPF: A sunscreen's effectiveness is measured by its sun protection factor (SPF). Depending on the active ingredient in the product being used, sunscreens absorb, reflect, or scatter ultraviolet rays away from the skin. The SPF indicates how long it will take for UVB rays to redden skin when using a sunscreen compared to how long skin would take to redden without the product. A sunscreen with an SPF of 15 will prevent reddening of the skin 15 times longer than without the sunscreen. For example, if someone starts to redden after 10 minutes without sunscreen, the use of an SPF 15 will prevent burning for about 2.5 hours. No SPF can block 100% of UV rays. The higher the SPF, the more protection you will receive from both UVA and UVB rays.

- SPF 15 screens 93% of the sun's UVB rays and some UVA rays.
- SPF 30 protects against 96%.
- SPF 50 blocks 98%.

Multi spectrum, broad spectrum, or UVA/UVB protection all indicate that some UVA protection is provided. The Skin Cancer Foundation supports that SPFs of 15 or higher are necessary for adequate protection. These sun protection filters fall into two categories: chemical and physical. Chemical filters form a thin, protective film on the surface of the skin, and through the chemical bonds, it *absorbs* the UV rays before they penetrate the skin. Some of the active ingredients that absorb UVB rays are octyl salicylate, octyl methoxycinnamate, and oxybenzone. The most commonly used ingredients in sunscreens that protect the skin from UVA rays include avobenzone, oxybenzone and butyl methoxydibenzoylmethane. The physical sunscreens that protect your skin from the sun by deflecting or blocking the sun's rays include titanium dioxide and zinc oxide. Some people who currently experience breakouts from mineral makeup and some sunscreens may find that titanium dioxide can be problematic for their skin. Zinc oxide, on the other hand, can be used on delicate skin. Most sunscreens contain a mixture of chemical and physical active ingredients.

You will want to make sure you're getting effective UVB as well as UVA coverage, so look for a sunscreen with an SPF of 15 or higher with a combination of the following UVA-screening ingredients: stabilized A avobenzone, ecamsule—also referred to as Mexoryl SX— oxybenzone, titanium dioxide, and zinc oxide. Just note that using multiple products that contain SPF ingredients does not add to your protection. For example, if your moisturizer contains SPF 30 and your face makeup contains SPF 20, the two do not add up to SPF 50.

Beside these basic skin-care routines, don't forget that what you eat also affects your skin says Inna Natkovitch a certified Medical Esthetician. Eating food high in essential fatty acids, such as fish, flaxseed oils, and olive oils, as well as food high in antioxidants will help to keep your skin looking healthier and younger. Don't forget to drink plenty of fluids; your skin needs to be well hydrated to prevent wrinkles.

Inna Natkovitch recommends treating yourself to a consultation with an esthetician, and getting facials done once a month if possible. Professional facials might help you to keep your pores clean. The application of rejuvenating masks to decrease wrinkle appearance and the massage that comes with the facial will stimulate blood flow to the face. If cost is an issue for you, try to find a beauty or aesthetic school in your area. They look for models for their students to work on to gain experience, and you would be given a guided facial under the instructor's supervision for free or for a reasonable price.

Besides a daily skin-care routine, you might need professional assistance with your skin, says Inna Natkovitch, and there are multiple options available to choose from. Here are some of them:

Microdermabrasion — This is a technique involving professional exfoliation of the skin performed by an aesthetician in a spa or salon. The outer layer of the skin is blasted with sand particles, which loosens the dead skin cells, which are then vacuumed out with all the dirt and oil on the skin. This helps to clean the pores and lighten the dark spots slightly. Microdermabrasion helps your skin feel cleaner and smoother. It is not painful, just mildly uncomfortable, and it doesn't require downtime. Microdermabrasion will reduce black heads and acne but will not reduce wrinkles.

Chemical Peels — Chemical peeling has become a popular procedure in the last 20 years. It is not a new invention of our century, though. Recipes for peeling were found in ancient Egyptian and Greek scripts. Our ancestors used different fruit and plant based juices with high acidic concentration to improve their skin texture. So what is a chemical peel? A chemical peel uses a chemical solution to smooth the texture of your skin by removing the damaged outer layers.

Although chemical peels are used mostly on the face, they can also be used to improve the skin on your neck, chest, and hands. Chemical peels are used to reduce fine lines and to treat wrinkles caused by sun damage, aging, and certain types of acne. Peels can also be used to decrease the appearance of freckles, age spots, and other pigmentation.

Chemical peels are available in different strengths and have different recovery periods. Some of them called lunch hour peels, are very mild, do not require a downtime, and show only a mild redness after the procedure. The skin will peel off gently, and this procedure can be performed once a month. The results are very mild, and it will take longer to see significant improvement.

Stronger peels require 1–2 weeks of downtime, but the results are more drastic and visible. Stronger peels should be performed by a certified medical professional such as a physician or a nurse practitioner. Peels might cause a higher risk for scar development if not applied correctly. Consult with your health care provider to decide which peel will work best on your skin type.

Botox — Richard Clark, a plastic surgeon from California, reported the cosmetic effects of botulinum toxin type A on wrinkles and was published in the journal *Plastic and Reconstructive Surgery* in 1989. Since then, it has been widely used for cosmetic and other medical conditions. Botox injections work by affecting the nerve ending in your face at the site of the injection. Affected nerve endings are paralyzed, and you will not be able to move your muscles, thus decreasing the appearance of your wrinkles.

Botox works great to improve the appearance of your frown lines, creases between the eyebrows, or wrinkles around the eyes. The results of a Botox injection could last from 4–6 months and may vary for different people. Botox is a fairly safe drug if administered correctly, but it does have some side effects.

The most common side effects include headaches, a cough, a runny nose, flu symptoms, dizziness, drowsiness, muscle stiffness, and neck pain. More serious side effect include difficulty swallowing, drooping eyelids, problems with vision, allergic reactions, chest pain, loss of bladder control, and a hoarse voice. It is important to choose an experienced health care provider to perform your Botox injections.

If not administered properly, Botox can cause a variety of side effects such as uneven brow lines and drooping eyelids on one side of the face. Botox should not be used by pregnant patients and patients with a history of neurological diseases; consult your health care provider to find out if Botox injections are safe for you.

Fillers — Fillers are rapidly becoming popular and are being widely used to smooth wrinkles and reshape the contours of the face. Made mostly from hyaluronic acid, these injectable medications can do wonders for your face. They are much cheaper and more affordable than a traditional facelift.

The only downside is that fillers last only 4–12 months as compared to a surgical facelift. Unlike Botox injections that relax the muscle under a wrinkle, injectable wrinkle fillers fill the line, crease, or area with one of several different substances. As a result, trouble spots nearly disappear.

Wrinkle fillers can also be used as "volumizers," plumping and lifting cheeks, jawlines, and temples; filling out thin lips; and plumping sagging hands. Some commonly used fillers are Belotero, Juvederm, Perlane, and Restylane.

Side effects from fillers are rare but can include redness, swelling, and bruising at the injection site. More serious side effects are blindness and death of the tissue at the injection site. Make sure to select a certified practitioner to inject your filler.

Treatment for Spider Veins

Spider veins are small, red, purple, and blue vessels that are easily visible through the skin. They are typically common on the legs and face. Varicose veins are raised, swollen blood vessels that usually develop in the legs, can be seen through the skin, and are larger than spider veins. Common causes for varicose and spider veins are heredity, occupations that involve a lot of standing, obesity, the hormonal influences of pregnancy, puberty, menopause, and the use of birth control pills.

Varicose veins require complex treatment usually performed by vascular surgeon. Spider veins, on the other hand, are not considered a significant health concern; they are aesthetically unpleasant and can be treated with laser treatment or sclerotherapy.

Sclerotherapy is a procedure that has been available since the 1930s. It involves an injection of a specific solution (usually highly concentrated salt or another detergent) directly into the vessel, which causes the vein to fade gradually in 3 to 6 weeks. This fairly safe procedure is simple to perform, relatively inexpensive, usually doesn't require anesthesia, and can be performed in the office.

Schedule a consultation with your health care provider and notify him or her if you are pregnant or taking medications such as blood thinners, aspirin, Motrin and other nonsteroidal anti-inflammatory medications, or herbal and dietary supplements. Before a procedure, don't apply any lotions to the area to be treated. Try to schedule your treatment before the weekend, and get some rest for several days after, avoiding any aerobic activity. Sclerotherapy solutions can be used for the veins of the body and should not be used on your face. Facial spider veins can be treated with a laser.

Laser Treatment is considered a safe and effective treatment option for spider veins on any body part including the face. A focused beam of light from the laser equipment is used to target a pigment in the blood, which heats up the small spider vein and destroys it in the process. The laser beam is very focused and precise, used to target a vessel only, and doesn't affect surrounding tissues.

The treated vein is gradually absorbed by the body and disappears in 4 to 6 weeks. Side effects include minor discomfort during the procedure and discoloration and blister formation of the treated area. The area to be treated should be free of lotions and creams before the procedure.

Avoiding the medications mentioned above for at least a week before laser treatment is also recommended.

Don't forget the rest of your body; it needs as much attention and care as your face. Following a healthy diet and exercise regimen will go a long way to help you feel and look better. Your outward appearance can say a lot about your personality, and looking your best on the outside can help you feel more confident and improve your self-esteem. So please find some time to spend on yourself and your appearance. Find time to be beautiful, to be confident, and to be yourself; you definitely deserve it.

PART III

HEALING YOUR SOUL

Chapter 10

FINDING YOUR TRUE SELF

"Waking up to who you are requires letting go of who you imagine yourself to be." Alan Watts

Finding your true self or actually being your true self is not an easy concept. We are influenced by our society and culture, which tells us what is considered the right thing to do, and often enough, we live our lives not the way we want but the way we are told or expected to live. Because of that, some of us deeply bury our own personal beliefs and dreams, hoping to fit in and function within expected norms. Being your true self sometimes is not acceptable in a particular environment.

As women, we have even more restrictions. Women tend to put family and children before their personal values, so finding our true selves oftentimes is put on the back burner and eventually becomes forgotten. I believe every woman has a right and deserves to have her values and beliefs valued and appreciated. Every woman deserves to have time to believe in herself and pursue her dreams and her passions. A question that follows this observation I often hear from other women is "I don't know what my true self is anymore. How can I rediscover it?" To answer that question, you need to look deep inside yourself and ask, "Who do I want to be?" rather than spend all your energy focusing on what other people around you—including your family and friends—expect or want you to be. You need to realize that you are unique; there is nobody else like you. You might not be perfect, but you are the best at being who YOU genuinely are. Life is a journey. In life, we learn how to improve and perfect our best self.

Shakti Gawain has an excellent quote, "*My true relationship is with myself – all others are simply mirrors of it.*" Once you find your true self, you are able to help other people to find themselves and be understanding, compassionate, and forgiving regarding other people's uniqueness. It is up to you to decide what makes you feel like your life is meaningful and fulfilling. Walter Anderson has a saying: "*Our lives improve only when we take chances – and the first and most difficult risk we can take is to be honest with ourselves.*" It is in your power to decide what your true self is and how you're going to live your life.

Believe In Yourself and Raise Your Self-Esteem

What is self-esteem? It is your own belief in yourself—the way you perceive, feel, and value yourself. Self-esteem plays a big role in your life. Self-esteem is a relationship that you have with yourself, and, in my opinion, it is the most important relationship you will ever have with anyone in this life. The esteem and respect you have for your own self impacts your relationships with the people around you. Before you can relate to others, you need to define your own values and beliefs as well as your outlook on life. This is all part of self-awareness, which also plays a role in self-esteem. Self-esteem is monumental in helping you to succeed in your undertakings and accomplish your goals in life. No wonder we all strive to increase our self-esteem; the question is, "How can I do it and do it correctly?" We women have a bad habit. Our inner voice constantly criticizes us by repeating, "I am too short or too tall," and "My nose is too big; my arms are too long; my lips are too thin . . ." The list goes on, and if we actually listen to these negative thoughts, we may start to believe them.

We beat ourselves up for decisions we have made. There are books written on how to get out from under these negative thoughts, termed "ANTS" by Dr. Daniel Amen, who wrote a wonderful book entitled *Change Your Brain, Change Your Life*. There is another book by Dr. L. Nehoc entitled *Illusion: Redefined*, which addresses who you are and who you are not. In it, the author cautions against defining yourself as what you have or have not accomplished. You are not your education, according to Dr. Nehoc. You are not the externals that money can buy. You are a spiritual being and need to own that.

The point is, if you believe you have a low self-esteem, that there is no hope for you, and success is out of your reach, you are wrong. Self-esteem is not a commodity that we are born with. It is an attitude we develop as we grow and move on with life. You have probably met women in your life that feel in control of their life and express self-confidence. They might seem to have a sense of self and purpose that comes across as high self-esteem and you might think that they are perfect. There is no such thing as perfection; every woman has her own shortcomings and flaws. The difference is that a woman with high self-esteem knows and understands herself well. She embraces her strengths, accepts her weaknesses, believes in herself, and emulates (without envy) those whom she chooses to follow. She chooses personal and professional mentors that guide her to be strong.

My grandmother had another saying: *"Stand tall with your head high, and believe in yourself. Everybody else will follow and believe in you as well."* She was right as usual; if you don't believe in yourself, then don't expect other people to believe in you. The good news is that self-esteem can be developed. It may not happen overnight; it may take time and patience – but it can be yours. Self-esteem is like a beautiful exotic flower; it needs to be nurtured and supported so it can bloom and flourish. To do that, you need to recognize and acknowledge your negative thoughts so you can stop or choose to ignore them. At the same time, you need to learn to accept and love yourself just the way you are.

Developing Your Self-Esteem

The first step in solving any problem is to assess the situation and gather information. To help you to develop and improve your self-esteem, you need to assess your strengths and weaknesses so you can know what areas should be worked on and improved. Take a piece of paper, and list what you believe your weaknesses are and what would like to improve; also list your strengths and what you believe your best qualities are. Dr. Nancy Iankowitz calls this "Writing Your Personality Resume." I am sure you can come up with at least ten qualities for each category. Now look at each one of your weaknesses, and ask yourself why you consider it a weakness. Are you comparing yourself to somebody else? How badly does it affect your life? Could you learn to accept it as is? If not, is there something that you can do about it?

It is not uncommon for women to focus on their self-identified weaknesses and complain about them continuously. As you know, complaining about your weaknesses is not going to change anything. You need to either learn how to live with them or do something to improve. For instance, if you are not good at cooking, and it affects your self-confidence, you could read cookbooks, watch cooking shows, or take cooking classes to improve your cooking skills. Yes, believe it or not, great chefs were not born cooking. They learned how to cook, and it took some time and practice. My grandmother used to say, *"There is no such thing as a weakness. Everybody is unique and is gifted with different characteristics; the best thing that you could do for yourself is to recognize your shortcomings and transform them into accomplishments."*

We often take for granted our unique skills and abilities and focus more on our shortcomings. For instance, you might say to yourself, *"I am just not good at telling stories and talking in front of people.*" It is okay. Maybe you are good at listening. People will respect you for that invaluable skill that not everybody has. So, instead of focusing on the things that you believe are negative, find things that you are good at. What I would like you to think about is a skill or an aptitude that you have that is natural to you; something you do easily and effortlessly. Is it something you think everyone can do? You might be wrong about that. It might be unique to you. Perhaps you are great at organizing things, or you might be excellent with numbers or good at writing. I am sure the list could be a very long one.

As a busy woman, I am sure you are excellent at multitasking. How else are you able to manage your life, family, work, AND have gotten this far in this book? What I would like to suggest is that you recognize and use your unique and special skills to your best advantage by using them to improve in areas where you are not as confident. Below are other things you can do to help increase your self-esteem.

Say Good-bye to Perfectionism

You think you are far from perfect? Guess what—nobody is perfect, so please let go of your perfectionism. We all have flaws, but we are all unique with our special talents, thoughts, and beliefs. Perfectionism can hold you back and prevent you from reaching your goals and accomplishing more in your life. You deserve to be and feel successful. Being a perfectionist takes a lot of time and energy. You might be busy focusing on getting every little detail exactly right, and you might miss the big picture and lose track of what is important. So, whenever you feel that you are spending too much time on a project, reflect on the bigger picture, and ask yourself what is really important. What is the worst thing that could happen if it isn't done to "perfection"? I'm not suggesting that you lower your standards. What I am suggesting is that you don't permit them to distract you from your goal. If particular details are crucial, then, of course, you need to do them a certain way; however, if whatever it is wouldn't matter, let's say, 6 months from now or a year down the line, then what is the energy being invested in, accomplishing the goal or distracting you from accomplishing it? Learn to do things the best way you can, and move on. And above all, accept yourself with your minor imperfections, put energy into self-reflection, growth, and self-improvement, and be patient because we are all works in progress.

Accept Your Mistakes the Positive Way

It is a great accomplishment, in my opinion, to learn to accept your mistakes and use them as learning experiences. Mistakes are inevitable in life. They are your steps in a road of learning and growth. So, instead of being negative and critical about yourself and your mistakes focus on what you learned from them and how much those mistakes helped you to grow and move on in life. Educate yourself, analyze the situation, and see what you've learned from that experience and what you might be able to do next time to avoid it. Be proud of yourself and your accomplishments even if those accomplishments were achieved through your mistakes.

Spend Time with Positive People

Stay away from negative people in your life—people who constantly criticize and belittle you no matter what you do. Negative people are like toxic substances that drain your energy as they try to bring you down. Spend time with positive people. Get yourself friends who respect and appreciate you for what you are. Surround yourself with happy, kind, understanding, and loving people who encourage and support you on your journey and who help you succeed, people who bring out the best in you.

Be Proud of Your Accomplishments

What do you consider your greatest accomplishments in life? Make a list of things and moments in your life that made you feel successful. Think back to those times; remember how proud you felt during those moments. What helped you to succeed on those occasions? Do you have knowledge or a special skill that helped you to succeed? You probably do; you just didn't realize it yet, right? What is this special skill? Could you use it for other things in your life? It is important to learn to be proud of your accomplishments regardless of whether they are big or small. It is equally important to reward yourself. Recognizing and rewarding your own accomplishments helps you to appreciate yourself more—and this builds your self-esteem.

Stop Comparing

Stephen Richards has an excellent quote: "*Stop comparing yourself with others. If they are good at something, you too are good at something else.*" What a true statement. How much time do we waste comparing ourselves to other people without realizing that we already have so much if not more than the person we are comparing ourselves to? And why do we most often compare ourselves to people who we believe are more fortunate than us? Why not reverse this thinking.

Whenever you meet a homeless person, let's say, compare that person to yourself, and acknowledge how blessed you are to have a roof over your head. It would be great if you stop comparing yourself to others completely and focus on your present self instead. Look at yourself today, and assess your past self. Do you want to change anything about yourself now for the future? What would make you more proud to be you? You are the best that you have. Spend your time and energy on improving yourself.

Chapter 11

THE HEALING POWER OF RELATIONSHIPS

"Personal relationships are the fertile soil from which all advancement, all success, all achievement in real life grows." Ben Stein

No matter how old we are or where we live, our lives constantly revolve around relationships. Our most painful and happiest moments in life are most likely connected to specific relationships. Relationships can often be complicated and frustrating and at the same time, elating and rewarding. Why are relationships so complicated and diverse? Of course, it is impossible to cover all the different aspects and nuances of relationships in one chapter of the book. What is more, no single recipe for a successful relationship exists that I know of and can share with you. We are all unique individuals with our special characteristics, complicated personalities, and interesting life stories. Carl Jung stated in his work: *"The meeting of two personalities is like the contact of two chemical substances: if there is any reaction, both are transformed."* In many instances, we may have no control of the situations and individuals that we interact with. We usually try to handle our relationships as we move on in life, which unfortunately is not always the best possible way. In this chapter, I would like to share some information that might help you to untangle some of the messy and frustrating aspects of your relationships and help you to learn how to create productive and meaningful relationships.

One of the most important aspects of all relationships is communication. Humans are social beings, and they interact with the world by receiving information, expressing themselves, and sharing information. Let's take a look what you can do to improve your communication skills.

The Art of Silence and Listening

Listening is an art, and those who have learned to be silent and listen have acquired a great skill. You might say, "How hard can that be? I always listen while other people are speaking." Yes, you might be silent and listening, but are you really paying attention to what is being said and what message that person is trying to convey? Are you trying to understand the other person's view, or are you busy forming in your head how you are going to respond to them? The majority of us do not finish listening to what other people are saying or try to understand and empathize with their point of view or their ideas. What we most likely do is start analyzing the conversation, and our thoughts start to wander, trying to find the best response. As a result, we often miss an important message that our companion was trying to convey. I have a colleague and a friend whom I have known over 15 years, and it is always amazing to watch her communicating with other people. People who barely know her are drawn to her and able to confide all their secrets and problems to her. She has an amazing ability to be silent and listen when you are trying to tell her something. She is present with you during a conversation and is able to understand you without inflicting her personal judgment or opinion on you. We all need someone to talk to and to be heard. If you have a friend or a family member who is a good listener, you probably admire and respect that individual, who is your go-to person when you need to confide in somebody. Wouldn't it be great if you learned that skill as well? It might take some practice on your part, but I believe it is a great skill to acquire. Good listening skills can help you to improve your relationships with your friends, family members, and colleagues. There are 2 excellent books written on this topic: *Just Listen: Discover the Secret to Getting Through to Absolutely Anyone* by Mark Goulston MD and *The Lost Art Of Listening: How Learning to Listen Can Improve Relationships* by Michael P. Nichols PhD. Both of these books offer great tips for mastering the art of silence and listening. Below are some examples that you can start practicing today:

- Keeping eye contact gives your companion the impression that you care about what they are trying to say.

- Monitor your thoughts while listening. Try to keep your thoughts from roaming around and focus on the conversation at hand.

- Do not interrupt. Let your companion finish his or her thoughts, and reply only if needed. Some people just need to talk and ventilate their feelings. They might not be necessary seeking your advice.

- Pay attention to nonverbal communication. Our words convey approximately 40–50% of our thoughts, and the rest of the message is communicated non-verbally. We use our tone of voice, our body movements, and our facial expressions to convey our messages. So it is very important to observe your companion and pay attention to what message is being conveyed. You should also remember your own body language. Are you relaxed and listening attentively to your companions, or are you constantly looking at your watch and thus giving your companions a message that you don't have time to listen to them?

- Express your understanding by encouraging your companion to continue the conversation. You could nod your head and say "yes" or "okay" to show that you understand the information given.

The Art of Dialogue and Communication

Effective communication is a crucial part of any relationship; it is a cornerstone for successful marriages, and it is a building block for an effective work environment. A common myth is that effective communications happens when people agree about everything and share similar thoughts and ideas. This is not necessarily the case. We all have different views and opinions on different topics, and it is okay to argue about them. It is how we argue that makes a big difference. What has a great impact on our relationships is how we handle conflicts and how effectively we handle our differences. Our conversations and the dialogue that follows can be stimulating or killing our relationships. They can be educational and bonding or pretentious and selfish. My grandmother had an excellent saying: "***Smart*** woman should know what to say. ***Wise*** woman should know how to say it and when to be silent." Her advice to me was to think carefully before saying anything and to answer these questions: What, When, and How?

For instance, before saying something, ask yourself, "Is ***What*** I am saying true? Does it make sense, and is it important and relevant to this conversation? Am I sharing valuable information, or am I gossiping about something or somebody just to feel more important? Is it kind, or am I going to hurt somebody by what I am saying?" Sometimes we might say things without thinking, intentionally or not, and it might hurt people around us. So think carefully, and weigh each word before it comes out. You won't be able to take it back.

When to say something is important as well. Who are the people around you? Are you having an appropriate conversation in this particular environment with these people? Is this the best time to say it, or should you wait for a better opportunity to verbalize your thoughts and intentions? You probably have met people in your life who speak out of turn, make inappropriate comments or jokes, or even worse, start preaching their ideas and believe at every opportunity. Preaching people truly believe in their philosophy and usually try to convince everybody that they are right. How do you feel about these people? Do you like to be in their company or find an excuse to leave the room as soon as you spot them? So, the next time you are engaged in a topic that you strongly believe in, pay attention to what you are saying and when you are saying it. Are you just sharing your thoughts and ideas, or are you preaching about them, trying to convince people that you are right? When you truly believe in something and behave accordingly, it will be noticed eventually, and people around you will be willingly asking your opinion and advice about that particular topic. It is very rewarding to share your believes with people who are willing and interested to listen and learn from you. Don't waste your time and energy sharing your beliefs and ideas when it is not wanted or appreciated.

How to say things correctly is a skill to be acquired as well. The tone and pitch of your voice and your verbal and nonverbal communication all play a role in how your message is received. Whether you are trying to resolve a conflict, are arguing about a project at work, or are simply trying to get your point across, it is important to stick to the facts and to avoid sounding overbearing and condescending. Delivering your message and opinion in a neutral, confident, and soft tone helps people to hear and respond to your message and not to the emotions that accompany an angry or tearful outburst. Using a negative tone when delivering your message causes people to become defensive and might cause them to automatically reject your idea. There is an excellent book titled *Crucial Conversations: Tools for Talking When Stakes Are High* by Kerry Patterson, Joseph Grenny, Ron McMillan, and Al Switzler, which offers great information and tools for improving your communication in different aspects of your life including conversations with your family, friends, and colleagues.

THE ART OF SUCCESSFUL RELATIONSHIPS

In previous chapter, we discussed the importance of having a healthy relationship with yourself. A woman who is confident thinks positive, loves and trusts herself, and is able to share her love and trust with others. Her positive thinking will help her to see positive qualities in other people and will help to form healthy and successful relationships. In this part of the chapter, I would like to cover how you, a busy woman, can share your positivity and confidence with others and learn to form loving, generous, and trusting relationships.

Relationships with Friends and Colleagues

How nice it would be if we worked and lived in a world of harmony and peace where everybody understood and respected each other, shared similar ideas, and had the same values. However, this is not the case. We live in a world that is far from perfect, and we meet people that might be completely different from us, have opposing views, and share different opinions from our own. The easiest solution would be to walk away from these people, but unfortunately, that might not always be possible.

So how do you deal with the people who might be driving you crazy? How would you behave if you met them at work or what would you do if you had neighbors who are not the nicest people to deal with? Well, the first order of business would probably be for you to realize that nobody is perfect, and you are not perfect as well. We all have our weaknesses and strengths. You need to understand that it is impossible for you to like everybody and realize that not everybody will like you either. This doesn't necessarily mean that the person you don't get along with is bad or wrong; it just means that the other person is different. My grandmother used to say, *"Two plus two is four, but so is three plus one and one plus three."* She also advised me to be patient and respectful of other people's ideas and beliefs.

People have a right to do things their own way and live their lives the way they feel is best for them. Wayne Dyer has a quote: *"Real magic in relationships means an absence of judgment of others."* You have a choice to react negatively to other people's differences and become upset every time you deal with them or to think about why this particular behavior upsets you. Could what you dislike in that person be something that you don't like in yourself? Confucius had an excellent quote: *"If I am walking with two other men, each of them will serve as my teacher. I will pick out the good points of the one and imitate them and the bad points of the other and correct them in myself."*

It is impossible to change all the people around you; your best choice is to work on changing yourself and the way you react to unpleasant situations and difficult people. I know this is not easy. How can you be nice to somebody who is inconsiderate, mean, and intentionally maligns your character? If you find yourself in this situation, do not react instinctively. Take a moment, and take a deep breath. Remember, if you retaliate and behave similar to this person, you automatically drop down to their level. There is a saying that I like very much: *"No matter how badly people treat you, never drop down to their level, just know you are better and walk away."* This might be difficult to do at the beginning, but once you set your mind to it, you will realize that being negative will bring only more negative things back. If you become rude and aggressive, you will receive anger and aggression back. Try to remain composed in any given situation, and you will keep your dignity and self-respect intact.

Here is another quote by Confucius: *"It is easy to hate and it is difficult to love. This is how the whole scheme of things works. All good things are difficult to achieve; and bad things are very easy to get."* Working on your own feelings and reactions takes a lot of time and effort, but I believe it is more worthwhile to spend all your energy on improving yourself rather than wasting that energy on negative reactions to the frustration that person is causing you. People will push your sensitive buttons only if you allow them to do so. If you refuse to be affected by other people's actions, there is nothing that they can do about it. Kindness attracts kindness, but I am not suggesting you to let other people mistreat and abuse you. There is an excellent quote by Zig Ziglar: *"Life is about balance: be kind but don't let people abuse you. Trust but don't be deceived; be content but never stop improving yourself."* If you are in a situation where you are being mistreated, keep calm and verbalize your feelings and thoughts while maintaining your decorum and dignity. The above-mentioned book, *"Crucial Conversations,"* devotes a whole chapter titled, "How to Stay in a Dialogue When You Are Angry, Scared or Hurt." As a last resort, if nothing else works, you can always walk away and keep your distance; remember, you have a choice.

Relationships with Family

Relationships with your family are probably even more complicated then relationships with your friends and colleagues. You can always change your job and stop seeing friends that you don't like anymore, but you can't choose a new family. So what is the best way to handle things in your family? Learn to be a little bit more patient and diplomatic with your family members; in most cases, they do have your best interest at heart. I have grown up in a culture that has to respect and listen to elders. This is not always easy to do as things are done differently nowadays. However, what I am realizing now as I am getting older is that even if times are changing, our parents do have a wealth of experience that they can share with us.

I have an incident in my life that thought me that lesson. When I delivered my first child, I was very anxious and inexperienced as is expected of any new mother. I was given a book on how to raise a child, which I followed to the letter. So, I rejected all the advice and help that was suggested to me by my mother and mother-in-law since it was different from what was in the book. You can imagine how stressful those days were for me. As the years passed by, and I delivered my second child,

I finally realized that in many instances, both my mother and mother in-law were right. I realized that they both raised 4 children each, and we came out fine, so I asked myself, why would I trust more in a book that was written by somebody I had never even met? If I had realized this sooner, I would have probably avoided a lot of the conflicts and arguments that I have had with them. I learned to be more diplomatic; I learned to compromise, and finally, I learned to give consideration to their advice, no matter what—they do have more experience than I do. Below are some other tips that you can consider when dealing with your family:

- Try not to criticize your family, especially the way your parents and in-laws raised their children. They probably did their best at the time, and it would be very painful for them to hear your negative comments. If you don't agree with their methods, you can use them to learn to avoid the same mistakes. Besides, you don't know how your own children will turn out yet, right?

- Be patient and more diplomatic when given advice. I know it might be very tiring to constantly hear how to do things correctly; however, believe it or not, in most cases, your family does have your best interest at heart. So be patient, say thank you, tell them you will consider their advice, and then do whatever you think is best.

- Try not to involve your family in your relationship conflicts with your partner. You eventually will resolve your conflict and make up; however, your family might not resolve things that easily. It might affect their attitude toward your partner or you in the future.

- Be more specific with your family regarding unexpected visits to your house. You might be polite and tell them that they are welcome at any time; however, in reality, you do want to be prepared for their visit. Sometimes, family members have an annoying tendency to show up at the worst time when your house is not clean or when you have nothing to eat at home. So discuss it beforehand with your family so you can come to an agreement about when the best time to visit is.

- Try not to complain about your partner to his family. Remember, they raised him, so he is their perfect child despite his flaws and shortcomings. Besides, you might hear in response, "If he is so bad, why did you choose him in the first place?"

Being considerate, tactful, and diplomatic will help you to achieve harmony and gain the respect of your family and your partner's family members. Having successful and healthy relationships with both families will prevent conflicts and strengthen and improve your relationship with your partner. In conclusion, I would like to share with you a quote from the Dalai Lama: *"A loving atmosphere in your home is the foundation for your life."*

FIFTY SHADES OF NOT SO GREAT

Have you heard about the popularity of the erotic romance novel series *Fifty Shades of Grey* by British author E. L. James? This erotic romance novel has taken America and the rest of the world by storm. It was translated into 52 languages, and over 125 million copies were sold worldwide. According to latest statistics, it was read by 86% of females, ages 14–88, and 14% of males; 55% of readers were married females. Despite the numbers of women reading this book, research studies conducted by various scientists showed that engaging in sexual activity is not a priority for many women. One sex survey published in *Time Magazine* indicated that women prefer food to sex; other surveys found that women may prefer to be more in touch with their sexuality but might not have the desire to do so. What is going on then? If women like to read and fantasize about sex, why do statistics suggest such a discrepancy? Why do so many women seem to have a decreased sexual drive and low libido?

This chapter will attempt to find answers to these questions. In considering the topic we will be addressing, let's begin by picturing this scenario of a busy woman's typical day:

She drops off her kids at school, rushes to work, and spends her day giving all she has to complete a project that is due. She gets back from work to pick up her kids from school and drop them off at a soccer or dance practice. Then, she does grocery shopping while kids are practicing and gets home (later) to prepare dinner and help with homework. After an entire day of giving herself to others, she is ready to go to bed and get some rest—then realizes that the laundry needs to be taken out of the dryer and folded and lunches need to be made for tomorrow. Finally, 45 minutes after she was ready to go to bed, she makes it to the bathroom to brush her own teeth, slips into pajamas, and then falls into bed. Sound familiar? Once she is finally in bed, her amorous partner is ready to have sex.

Let's just take a closer look at this situation: what is going through *her* mind? How does she feel? What mood is *she* in? Even though she might have read a chapter of a sizzling novel during her 12-minute lunch break, sex is probably the last thing on her mind after a full day at work and selfless mothering with her kids. Clearly, she is so stressed and tired by the time she gets to bed that having sex is the last thing on her mind. Why? Perhaps, at that moment, she just has nothing left to give her partner. Maybe she could use a back rub or a foot massage, but she certainly has no energy to return the favor.

If this is a familiar scenario in your life, you might think the easiest solution would be to get some rest to renew your sexual appetite. Maybe it would . . . but when? During a vacation? Maybe. But in general, getting more quality sleep is unfortunately not as simple as it sounds. There might be different or additional reasons why your sex life is not as exciting as you want it to be. There are various psychological and physiological factors that might contribute to a low sex drive. Below is the list of the most common ones:

Hormonal imbalances. Testosterone, estrogen, and progesterone are three (3) important hormones needed for your sexual health:

Testosterone is a male sex hormone produced in women in smaller amounts than in men by the ovaries and adrenal glands. It is responsible for sexual desire and increased sensitivity in the vagina and clitoris during intercourse.

Estrogen is responsible in increasing the blood flow to the genital area and providing lubrication during intercourse.

Progesterone, called a "feel good hormone," is increased during ovulation and causes an increased sex drive.

Other hormones that might affect your libido are prolactin, the thyroid and adrenal gland hormones discussed previously. If these hormones are out of balance for any reason, they have a great impact on lowering your libido.

Physiological factors such as poor nutrition, lack of sleep, and lack of exercise can all affect your sex drive.

- Poor nutrition related to a diet low in healthful fats and high in simple sugars might cause insulin resistance and decrease the production of sex hormones.
- Lack of sleep increases physiological stress to your body as it increases cortisol levels and decreases the production of sex hormones.
- A regular exercise regimen increases testosterone levels, which are responsible for your sex drive, while a sedentary lifestyle decreases testosterone levels.

Psychological factors including negative attitudes about sex, past unpleasant experiences with sex (such as abuse), a poor body image, low self-esteem or a history of depression in one of the partners are all factors that may greatly impact your sex life and subconsciously cause aversion to sex and create a low libido.

Emotional factors play an important role as well. The brain is considered the biggest sex organ for women. So, any emotional issues such as unresolved conflicts between partners, a lack of communication of sexual needs, increased emotional stress at work or with family members, difficulty communicating with a partner, and infidelity of a partner may all potentially have a negative impact on your sex drive.

Medications such as antidepressants, birth control pills, pain medications (i.e. opiates), and blood pressure medications are known to cause side effects such as a decreased libido.

Dyspareunia or pain during intercourse results from a decline in estrogen levels especially during the premenopausal and menopausal years. This decline causes physical changes in the genital region. The tissue lining the vagina and vulva becomes thin, dry, and tight. This often leads to pain and discomfort during intercourse. If you experience this, speak with your gynecologist for assistance. Help is available.

Getting Your Sexual Life Back

If you are having problems with your sex drive, the first order of business is to find out the cause. Is the problem related to hormonal imbalances, medications, or any emotional or psychological issues that need to be resolved? Talk to your health care provider if you believe your symptoms are side effects of your medications, and ask if you could be prescribed a different medication. You might need to visit a psychologist or a therapist to get assistance to help you resolve any psychological or emotional traumas from the past that are affecting your sex life.

For information related to testing and treatment for hormonal imbalances, refer to the previous chapters where these issues are addressed. This book also offers a wealth of information on healthy lifestyles, proper dieting, exercises, and sleep habits, which, if followed, might help to balance your hormones as well. Sex can be a wonderful and important part of your life. Feeling sexy and sensual has a profound effect on every woman, increasing your self-esteem and feelings of desirability as well as improving your mood and outlook on life. An active sex life may also be of benefit to your overall health. See the list below:

Stress reduction — Oxytocin and endorphins released during sex have a great effect on decreasing your stress levels. This "feel-good" hormone affects pleasure centers in your brain and helps you to relax and calm your mind.

Promotes sleep — The pleasant relaxation that you feel after having sex is due to oxytocin and prolactin being released, both of which have a calming effect that helps you to sleep better after satisfying lovemaking.

Boosts your immune system — Recent research studies revealed that people who had sex regularly had higher levels of antibodies called immunoglobulin A (IgA). IgA boosts your immune system and helps you to fight infections.

Sex as an exercise — We already mentioned that sexercise can be counted as a cardio workout and can help you burn up to 300 calories, depending on how long and vigorously you participate. So if you didn't have time to exercise during the day, you can still make it up in bed at night.

Bladder control — Regular intercourse is similar to performing Kegel exercises, which help to strengthen and tone your pelvic muscles. Stronger pelvic muscles help to maintain bladder control and prevent incontinence.

Enhances glowing skin — Have you ever wondered why women experience "after-sex glow"? First, during intercourse, there is an increased circulation of blood to body tissues, which helps to oxygenate the skin cells and promote skin regeneration. Second, regular sexual activity increases the production and release of hormones such as estrogen and DHEA (dehydroepiandrosterone), which are responsible for keeping the body young and beautiful.

Besides visiting your health care practitioner and balancing your hormones, there are a lot of other things that you could do to reawaken your sex drive. Here are some examples:

Talk to your partner. It is a well-known fact that we women do like to talk, but unfortunately, we do not do so in the bedroom. Many research studies found a lack of communication between partners is one of the most common causes of a low sex drive in women. Your partner is not a mind reader, so please do teach, coach, and tell him what you want and what gives you pleasure. The majority of men state that they are more than willing to pleasure their partners if only they knew how to do it.

Be open to new exploration. It is not uncommon for couples who have lived together for several years to have their sex life become perfunctory or boring. Sometimes it can help to spice it up a little bit. Try something new. Choose a different place in the house where you have never done it before, or maybe try a different pose. As you and your partner move on through your life and change, your sexual needs might change as well. Talk to your partner, and add variety to your sexual routine. Enjoy a mutual journey of intimacy and exploration. When sex is done with respect, love, and mutual interest, it can enhance your relationship on many levels.

Keep intimacy ongoing. Our busy lives and a long list of responsibilities often keep us preoccupied, and we spend less and less time with each other. It is important for couples to keep intimacy going. Perhaps you can give each other a hug and a kiss in the morning or soft touch and cuddling while watching TV in the evening. Try to let go of your responsibilities during these moments and relax during sex, opting to deal with the responsibilities later.

Have morning sex. If a busy life prevents you from having sex at night, try it in the morning. Your cortisol levels are naturally elevated in the morning, so you should have enough energy to enjoy sex. You don't necessarily need a lot of time; you might enjoy a quick sexual encounter with your partner for 10–15 minutes. This offers benefits such as a feeling of satisfaction from your mutually loving experience as well as a broad smile, good mood, and boost of energy for the rest of the day.

Spice it up. Some couples watch erotic movies to add a little spice to their sex lives, but if it is something against your nature, you can choose any type of movie, including a thriller. Adrenalin produced during a fight or flight response might have similar effects on your arousal because both of these hormones are produced in the same part of the brain.

Reawaken your sexuality. A majority of women require longer sexual warm-ups than men do. So help your partner, and get yourself in the right mood during the day. One way to do this is to wear sexy and sensual underwear that you like under your working clothes during the day. This may help you to feel more sensual and release your "feel-good" hormone oxytocin, which causes you to experience those tingling and pleasurable sensations when you are aroused.

Use lubrication. Menopause, birth control pills, and breastfeeding can all contribute to vaginal dryness and discomfort. To decrease the pain and discomfort caused by vaginal dryness you might benefit by using one of the water-based lubricants stocked in pharmacies, such as K-Y jelly or other brands. If you are experiencing more serious issues such as vaginal tearing or bleeding during penetration, seek help from a specialized health care provider, and ask if you might benefit from a vaginal renewal program. You can obtain more information regarding a vaginal renewal program at www.sexualityresources.com

Take supplements. Ask your health care provider if you might benefit from a supplement called ArginMax. This product contains an herbal combination of ginseng, L-arginine, ginko biloba, damiana, multivitamins, and minerals, which might help to improve your libido. Another herbal blend to consider is Zestra—a topical blend of oils and extracts containing borage seed oil, evening primrose oil, angelica extract, coleus extract, vitamin C, and vitamin E. Zestra has been shown to increase sexual sensations, arousal, and pleasure when applied topically to the genital area.

Visit a sex boutique. Explore different options, including sexual aids, and discuss these with your partner. If you feel uncomfortable visiting a sex boutique, there are many online stores that offer a wide variety of sex toys including Ben Wa Balls, French ticklers, scented oils, and lubricants.

Initiate sex with your partner. Most men enjoy it when their partners initiate sex; however, depending on your cultural values and your upbringing, initiating sex yourself might not be considered "lady-like" behavior. Some women also might be afraid to hear "no" as this type of rejection frightens them for a variety of reasons. If this is the case with you, and you don't want a direct approach, you might use other subtle ways such as sexting to your partner during the day, giving him a present of sexy lingerie for yourself, or leaving a piece of your sexy underwear in his car for him to find. These things might help you and your partner to build anticipation, so use your imagination.

Improving your relationship with your partner might also help you to improve your sex life. After living together for some time, many couples gradually grow apart. As personal interest in each other dwindles down, so does sexual desire. So it might help to reinvent your relationship from time to time. Love in a relationship is a living and real element. It needs to be nurtured and supported to grow. If you don't work on it, it will die out. You don't have to necessarily do any big gestures; you can strengthen your relationship with small steps on daily basis. Here are some examples:

- Giving compliments to each other and being affectionate helps to foster the feelings of love in your relationship.

- Bring kindness and generosity into your relationships, and leave criticism and hostility behind. Contempt and criticism of the partner damage and kill the love in a relationship, while generosity and kindness help to reciprocate those feelings and make each partner feel cared about and loved.

- Share joy, and celebrate each other's accomplishments—this will help to bring you both closer and provide an opportunity to bond together.

- Learn to accept and forgive each other's weaknesses. Holding grudges and pointing blaming fingers will eventually destroy your feelings of love. Being generous and giving will help to evoke your loving feelings and keep the romance and love ongoing.

- Learn to say, "I am sorry" and to acknowledge your mistakes. In an argument, try to put yourself in your partner's shoes, and try to understand his point of view.

- Choose your arguments wisely—not all the things are worth fighting for; life is short, and you have a choice whether to live in harmony and peace or not. If you put some effort in changing your own behavior, your partner might decide to follow your example.

- Try doing thoughtful things for your partner. You probably know what things make your partner happy. With a small effort on your part, you can bring that happiness into his life, and you will see that your thoughtfulness will be reciprocated and rewarded.

There are also many books to help you on your journey to reclaim your sexuality and improve your relationship. One of the oldest is probably the Kama Sutra—an ancient marriage manual from India. Some other books to read are *Reclaiming Desire* by Andrew Goldstein, M.D. and Marianne Brandon, PhD, *Reclaiming Your Sexual Self* by Kathryn Hall, and *The Heart of Desire* by Stella Resnick, PhD.

Of course, there are many more other good books and resources available, and you are welcome to explore them all. Sex and intimacy are an amazing and a wonderful part of life when they are a dance of love and respect between partners who are full of passion. This rhythmic connection is enhanced when there is a sacred, spiritual union—all of which you deserve to experience and enjoy.

PART IV

SELF-TRANSFORMATION

Chapter 12

TRANSFORMING YOUR LIFESTYLE

"Transformation is not a future event. It's a present day activity."
Jillian Michaels

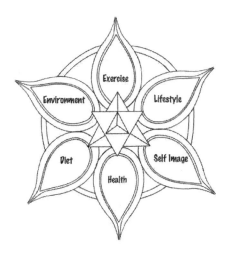

Transforming Flower of Wellness

This part of the book is about change. You now have the tools to help you transform and heal yourself. I am hoping that since you've arrived at this point, you have probably given serious thought—and might have even already begun—to make the changes in your life that are meaningful to you. At least, that is my assumption. Congratulations! We are ready to continue to the next steps. Now you will read step by step instructions designed to help you to continue implementing the changes you may have already begun making to your diet, exercise habits, lifestyle, self-image, environment, and your health. It is natural to feel overwhelmed at first since there is so much new information to absorb and so many things that need to be considered. Please don't get discouraged. Do one thing at the time. Implement the changes gradually, and decide which changes you agree with and want to keep for the rest of your life. As you move through this journey of transformation, celebrate and feel good about each accomplishment, regardless of how big or small it might seem right now. Remember: growth is a lifetime journey. Time is immaterial. Transformation is not a short-term goal, but rather, a lifelong adventure. This book is a guide to point you in the right direction. It is accompanying you at the beginning of your journey, which is your personal path to a healthier and happier you. Deepak Chopra has an excellent quote: *"I can affect change by transforming the only thing that I ever had control over in the first place and that is myself."* I am confident that since you've read this far, you are ready—so let's get started.

Being busy is challenging and sometimes frustrating. You might feel, at times, that you need to clone several of you in order to accomplish all that is on your plate. There are days you wish you had 4 arms instead of 2, two heads instead of one, and subdivisions within the hours of the day to permit you to simultaneously accomplish career-centered tasks and home related responsibilities all before even considering taking time for yourself. There are days you might find yourself wishing you could just freeze the clock for 30 minutes.

Sounds familiar, doesn't it? I was once told that if your plate is too heavy, take something off it. Sounds easy, but I can't pass this advice along because it is simply not always possible to choose who or what to "remove," and just thinking about having to choose can create stress. And yet, what do we busy women tend to take off our plate? We neglect ourselves. Our own needs are usually the first to go. Then sometimes, the house doesn't get cleaned. Sometimes, our relationship with our partner doesn't get the attention it deserves. Healthy boundary setting is necessary in order to find quality time for ourselves so that we have patience and attention along with all the necessary energy to offer to everyone and everything else on our plate—including our children and our aging parents.

Sometimes, we are able to afford to stop working and stay home to raise the kids—but this is more than likely not the scenario. If you enjoy your work or going to school because these things are as much a part of you as all the other things you have on your plate, perhaps rearranging the plate is in order. Everything has a time and place.

Did you ever begin to clean your kids' closet only to discover that everything was shoved in? Did you wonder how your children were ever able to find anything in that cluttered mess? The closet looked full and ready to burst, with no space for anything new. After spending a half hour folding and rearranging everything—voila!—finally, you established order and enough space to add more items.

I would like you to try the same thing with your stressful, overflowing, and complicated life. Take a piece of paper and try to plot your activities for a week. I would like you to list all your activities every day by the hour. Now, look at your schedule, and see if there are things that you could rearrange or move around to make your day look more organized. Is there anything that you could do to find some time for yourself? And keep in mind that getting up earlier in the morning or going to bed later are not options—we've already discussed the importance of getting enough quality sleep for your health and well-being. Twenty-four hours is all you have during the day, so don't waste even a minute of it.

To help you to get more organized, I suggest you get a planner. There is an excellent website www.theconfidentmom.com that offers a great weekly household planner for moms. They also offer a toolkit for purchase to help you to get organized. If you are not a mother yet, check out this great website www.thebusywoman.com, which offers a variety of daily, weekly and monthly planners for busy women. There are also different electronic apps on the market, such as Motivated Moms, which offer excellent organizational tools. Do some research, and choose what will work best for you. You can use your planner to help you to organize your work, home, personal routine, and tasks.

List things to be done by priority for today, this week, this month, and this year. Leave some room for unexpected things and events, and always have a plan B if possible. Use your calendar to list important events, such as birthdays, holiday dinners, and your children's recitals and sport practice. Don't forget to write down the things you would like to accomplish for yourself.

When you finish writing your list of chores, examine it, and see if some of them could be delegated to your family, friends, or colleagues at work. Remember, you don't have to do everything yourself, and not everything needs to be done at once or perfectly. Does everything have to be "your way" or is there room for compromise so that others can pitch in? Do you need to be a Superwoman?

One of the things that helped me with my busy life of working full time, going to school, and being a mom was to assign chores to my children and make them responsible for their self-care. For instance, to avoid a mad dash in the morning, I realized that looking for lost homework and socks at the last minute was time consuming and a time waster. To address this, my kids began to prepare their book bags, lunchbox, and their clothes the night before, so in the morning, everything was ready to go.

Another important task that my kids now help with is menu planning for the week. We put together a weekly menu plan with their favorite food listed on it, and then do grocery shopping to get what we needed for that week. My kids also help me with household chores, including folding the laundry, setting the table, cleaning their own rooms before bedtime, and making their beds in the morning. It might not seem like much, but when you are busy, every minute counts.

So once you get organized, the time is right to declutter your life and transform yourself. The first step is to assess your lifestyle and list things that you would like to change. Then, review that list and prioritize the tasks/desires. Ask yourself what you think needs to be changed first, what could be postponed until later, and if you can, estimate the time it would take to change. If your list of things is long, cross out some of goals for now so you don't get overwhelmed. Change is not easy and needs your time and commitment to be successful. I would advise you to start with something easy, something that would not require a lot of time and effort to succeed and could be done gradually. Set a plan of action to plan and prepare for a change. When you feel out of control or not prepared, it is tempting to fall back into old patterns, so do try to make goals and plans that are sustainable. This is the key to positive change. Short- and long-term goals are important. Here is a sample plan of action:

a. Changing your environment
b. Changing your diet
c. Getting fit and exercising
d. Changing your appearance
e. Changing your relationship

Your list can be shorter or longer, and the priority of the things to be changed is up to you as well. Choose one goal for a week, a month, or even for just a day, and start walking down the path to a healthier and happier you.

Chapter 13

TRANSFORMING YOUR ENVIRONMENT

"If you focus on results you will never change. If you focus on change, you will get results." Jack Dixon

Okay, so you have a list of things that need to be changed, and you are ready to start your transformation, but you aren't certain exactly where to begin. Well, the first step is to do an assessment, which is like going on a treasure hunt.

Get a pad of paper and pen so that you can take down notes as you walk through your home assessing everything with a critical eye. Write down all the problem areas and what needs to be done. Room by room, look around to decide what you treasure and what you are willing to part with. What deserves to be kept? What needs to be thrown away? What needs to stay as it is because it functions well, and what should be changed or improved upon to function better? What do you love and cherish? What is weighing you down?

This task is similar to weeding a garden – but you are working on the garden of your life. Check your bathroom to see if you need to change the type of soap, shampoo, or toothpaste that you use. Check your kitchen. Is it clean, functional, and stoked with healthy foods? What kinds of utensils do you use? Are they safe and clean? Check all the bedrooms in your home. Are they comfortable and conducive to sleeping? Do they actually look like bedrooms, or are they full of electronics such as computers, TV, phones, or a PlayStation? Is there clutter? Are books, magazines, or papers piled up? Are projects or homework half done? Check your closet and your makeup station. Do you need to change things there as well? While you assess your environment, also take a look at what could be improved upon or rearranged. Can you find a time for your exercise routine? Is there a special quiet place to meditate and have some "me time"?

Once you have your list, I don't want you to throw anything out—yet. A very common mistake people make is to throw out old items before replacing them. Since you don't know yet what new and healthy things you might need or where to get them, I would like you to do some research. Below is the list of things that need to be changed in your environment.

Water — Public tap water is unfortunately chlorinated and treated with fluoride, bromide, and over 200 other chemicals. Look into buying a home purifying water system for your house. If buying the whole system is not an option for you at present, buy a kitchen sink filter, or use bottled water for drinking and cooking.

Air — Everybody likes to have a clean and nice smell to their house and environment. Do you love those vanilla or apple-cinnamon candles or orange and spice air fresheners? I love them too, but they are not safe; they are not made from fresh apples or oranges and are actually made from harmful chemicals such as benzene, which can cause allergic reactions and a list of other unhealthy side effects. So get an air filter in your house, and use essential oil based alternatives for pleasant aromas in your home environment.

Household cleaners — Yes our house needs to be cleaned, and if you have kids or pets, your home probably needs cleaning more than those who don't. Choose your household cleaners carefully. Most products on the market are filled with dangerous petrochemicals, which are harmful if ingested or inhaled. There are many alternatives available such as Seventh Generation, Earth Friendly Products, and Whole Earth foods.

Kitchenware — You have probably heard of BPA—Bisphenol-A. It is a chemical used in plastic products, which was found to be very toxic through exposure. Be mindful of this, and avoid plastic utensils, storage containers, water bottles, and other plastic kitchen accessories; do not heat your food in a plastic container. Heating releases chemicals right into the food you eat. Healthy alternatives to using plastic are glass, stainless steel, silver, and wood products.

Cookware — Ceramic, glass, cast iron, stainless steel, and stoneware are rapidly making a comeback. We are returning to their use, choosing these over nonstick cookware, and with good reason. Nonstick pans and pots have PFOA—perfluorooctanoic acid, a chemical that can cause a list of health problems including cancer and infertility.

Skin-Care and Hygiene products — Look through your bathroom and cosmetics cabinets, and throw away anything that contains parabens, dyes, lead, SLS (sodium laurel sulfates), benzoyl peroxide, DEA (diethanolamine), DMDM hydantoin (formaldehyde releaser), synthetic colors and pigments, phthalates, and triclosan. Check the Environmental Working Group website (www.ewg.org)_for a full list of chemicals to avoid and safer alternatives for cosmetic products.

Food — The food that you eat should also be inspected and chosen carefully. Unfortunately, in America, we don't always get the best quality food: fruits and vegetables are treated with pesticides and are genetically modified; animal products are filled with hormones and antibiotics; supermarkets are filled with products containing artificial sweeteners, coloring, preservatives, modified hydrogenated oils, and other chemicals that are impossible to pronounce or spell. How do you know what is healthy to eat? The Environmental Working Group has a list called "The Dirty Dozen," which includes a list of fruits and vegetables that have the highest content of pesticides and should be bought organic. They also have a list of products called "Clean 15," which lists products that are safe to eat and have the least amount of chemicals if grown conventionally. As a general rule, get into the habit of reading labels on the food you buy. The fewer ingredients it has, the better it is for you. Look for products that are free of chemicals, artificial coloring, flavors, sweeteners, hydrogenated oils, shortening, and high fructose corn syrup. If possible, buy products that are organic and GMO free.

This list is not complete. There is more, but don't get discouraged; there is hope. As time goes on and more research is done on the harmful effects of our environment on our health, more and more products are being banned by the government. For now, be your own guide. Start by slowly changing and experimenting with products one by one. It might take a while before you find a product that you like and enjoy and is also healthy and safe for you and your family. Be patient, and enjoy your treasure hunt. You are definitely worth it.

Chapter 14

TRANSFORMING YOUR SELF-IMAGE

"A strong positive self-image is the best possible preparation for success in life."
Dr. Joyce Brothers

This book is all about transforming your "self" to become a better **you**—inside and out. In this chapter, I will talk about self-image, which is connected directly to self-confidence.

In order to have a strong and positive self-image, you need to believe in yourself. Your mind and the way you feel deep inside play a major role in how you look. This book began with a "Mind" chapter because your mindset plays the most important role in everything that you do and feel. If you have a mindset that you are a self-confident and beautiful woman, your work on your self-image is halfway done. You now need to apply the finishing touches so you can present that self-confident, gorgeous woman to all who view you from the outside. Style is not inherited, and you are not born with it. My first career choice was in fashion design, and I had the pleasure of spending several years of my life in the fashion industry. I learned a lot about style and fashion, which helped me to develop my own sense of style. I also taught my clients to develop their own sense of style, which was congruent with their personality and beliefs. This ability is not as difficult as it sounds, and it can be learned. You will learn how to develop your own, unique sense of style.

In previous chapters, we discussed how to boost self-esteem and change one's lifestyle. We also addressed issues about your environment, relationships, and nutrition to help you to improve your strength and health. This chapter will cover things you need to know in order to present your best self from the outside. We will discuss how to choose your style and dress and how to apply makeup to emphasize your individuality and uniqueness. You might already have your own personal style of dressing as well as your own defined self-image. In fact, you may be very comfortable with all you are currently doing. If so, congratulations! It is wonderfully inspiring when self-image and self-confidence walk hand in hand.

If, however, you believe you don't know yet what your self-image and style should be, that is also fine as this chapter is meant for you. I am hoping the information in this chapter will help you to choose a self-image that will enhance your self-confidence and emphasize the best in you.

DRESSING FOR SUCCESS

First impressions do count. As you can imagine, we don't get a second chance to make a first impression. So dressing for success means we strive to make a good first impression. Before I go into detail about how to dress for success, I will discuss different styles and ways of dressing. So what do the words "stylish" and "beautiful" really mean? These questions have been asked by women for thousands of years, and depending on the century and culture, there are—as you can imagine—a variety of answers. There is the mysterious smile of Mona Lisa, the elegance and charm of Princess Diana, the sensuality and sex appeal of Marylyn Monroe, as well as the class and elegance of Grace Kelly and Audrey Hepburn. The list goes on and on.

Each of these ladies was different. Each had her own unique sense of style and fashion, and each was beautiful in her own way. So, to help you to find your own style to enhance and express your personal self-image, you first need to realize that you are unique. Next, you need to decide what style suits you best and makes you feel comfortable. Do you prefer looking elegant, classy, or sexy? Do you prefer to look feminine, unconventional, sensual, or more sophisticated and understated? There is no right or wrong answer here; you need to choose what suits you best.

When you are wearing an outfit that you like, it makes you feel beautiful and confident, which will show in your posture and attitude. If you wear an outfit that you don't like, you will feel uncomfortable, and your displeasure will be evident in your facial expression, vibrations, and behavior. You don't have to choose one particular style and stick to it. You may choose to wear a sophisticated business suit to work and a feminine sensual dress to a party, for example. True success in looking great is to wear clothes that are appropriate for the occasion and your body shape.

Appropriate for the Occasion

It goes without saying that any outfit will look great if it is appropriate for the occasion it is worn to. Even though there are no special rules written anywhere, it is important to dress appropriately as defined by the occasion, place, and time of day. That is, you would not wear a ball gown to go shopping or yoga pants to a wedding—at least, that would not be the norm. Am I right?

When you dress for an occasion, choose a style that you are comfortable with and that is unique to you. Do not let fashion statements and expensive logos guide you if you do not believe in them. When invited to a celebration—a birthday party or wedding, for example—make it a habit to ask the hostess how formal your dress should be, and where the event will take place. You will need to plan your outfit accordingly. For instance, if a birthday celebration is planned outside in the garden or at the beach, wearing stiletto sandals and a swing skirt probably would not be the best choices.

If the event is a wedding celebration at a restaurant, inquire how formal is it and if the hostess's family observes any religious tradition. This approach will help you to avoid any embarrassment and will ensure that you pay proper respect to the occasion, especially if you might have been inclined to wear a color or style that doesn't honor the religious traditions.

I learned the lesson above the hard way—from personal experience. I attended a Jewish wedding but didn't realize that it was a religious orthodox ceremony. I wore a short (above the knee) dress, and, in case you are unfamiliar with the culture, modesty is a high priority. Women are expected to have covered shoulders, and, usually, dresses are mid-calf. You can just imagine how embarrassing this experience was, and I'm certain you can understand why I spent the entire wedding hiding my legs beneath the table, grateful that at least my dress had long sleeves.

If you are planning to attend a formal business meeting or a dinner, choose an outfit that emphasizes your sophistication and independence. It is best to stick with elegance and simplicity. Choose solid colors, avoid flashy or ruffled shirts, leather, or above-the-knee skirts, and keep your jewelry to a minimum. Choose clothing that is appropriate to your size. Avoid squeezing into clothes that are tight. Edith Head has an excellent quote: *"A dress should be tight enough to show you're a woman and loose enough to prove you're a lady."* Straining buttons and sliding up skirts make one appear unkempt and disheveled; thus, avoid them. Wear clothes that are comfortable and that do not restrict your movement. Makeup and nail color should be neutral, and they should complement your features. Bright colors are distracting—avoid wearing bright eyeshadow and lipstick to a business meeting; keep them for evening occasions.

Appropriate for Your Body Shape

Coco Chanel once stated, *"Fashion is architecture; it is a matter of proportions."* She was absolutely right. Women who have the same height and weight might have different body shapes. Have you ever experienced seeing a gorgeous dress on another woman, but when you tried it on, discovered it just didn't look right? Having the ability to choose an appropriate style for yourself involves first knowing your body type. What shape are you? Body shapes are categorized as follows: **pear, apple, hourglass, rectangle, and triangle.** Each shape has its advantages and disadvantages, and each has characteristics to maximize and minimize. The trick is to choose outfits that help you to make the most of your features and characteristics. Another way to state it is that your goal is to create an illusion of proportion.

Body Shapes

Pear — Your hips are the widest part of your body, and your shoulders are narrow, so the goal of your chosen outfit would be to balance and elongate your figure by enhancing your upper body. Focus on wearing light colored tops and dresses that add volume to your shoulders and darker shades of skirts and pants to slim down your hips. Your best choice for skirts and dresses would be an A-line or a fit and flare style, which tend to accentuate the waist and hide wide hips. Wearing shoes with heels will help to elongate your body as well.

Apple — Your hips are slim and your middle is the widest part of your body. To balance and enhance the proportions of your body type, you would need to wear clothes to slim your midsection and accentuate your legs and shoulders. A-line shape dresses and skirts work best. Wear them with a belt to slim down your waist. Choose clothes with solid colors or vertical stripes to slim and elongate your body.

Hourglass — Your body is curvy with well-shaped hips, a slim waist, and a voluptuous bust. Your body shape is the easiest to dress; however, you need to focus on doing it right to look elegant and classy. You can wear wrap dresses and belted jackets to accentuate your slim waist. Pencil skirts look best on you. Pair them with cropped or scooped neck tops.

Rectangle — Your body shape is straight and has minimal curves. Your outfits need to focus on adding curves to your body while slimming your waist. Wear ruffled tops to enlarge your bust. Skirts with a visible waist and pleats or lace add volume to your hips. Choose high waist and boot cut pants to add curves to your hips.

Inverted triangle — Your body has wider shoulders and slim hips, resembling a more masculine body shape. Your outfits should focus on slimming your upper body and adding curves to your hips. Your best choices include darker tops and lighter bottoms. Avoid ruffled tops and pencil skirts. A-line and fit and flare skirts work best to add volume to the hips and slim your waist.

You can also use shaping undergarments to help to temporarily alter your body shape. There are a wide variety of slimming girdles to smooth your thighs and stomach and padded panties to add shape to your buttocks. There is also hip padding and pushup bras for anyone who needs them. It is important to remember to choose the right undergarment and be sure it fits correctly. Stores such as Victoria's Secret offer services to help you to fit your bra correctly. You may also do it at home yourself. All you need is a measuring tape.

To choose an appropriate size for your bra, first measure your band size by running a tape measure around your body fairly snug underneath your breast; write down this number in inches —for example, 30 or 34 inches. This is your bra band size. To determine your bra cup size, measure around your chest with the tape over the fullest part of your breast. To figure out your cup size, subtract your band measurement from your cup measurement; this number difference is what determines your cup size:

1 inch (2.5 cm) = A
2 inches (5 cm) = B
3 inches (7.5 cm) = C
4 inches (10 cm) = D
5 inches (12.5 cm) = DD
6 inches (15 cm) = DDD
7 inches (18 cm) = DDDD/F
8 inches (20.5) = G/H
9 inches (23 cm) = I/J
10 inches (25.5 cm) = J

If you are still not sure you are wearing the right bra, look at your bra now. Does your bra band fit your chest snuggly, or is it riding up between your shoulder blades? Do your shoulder straps stay in place, or do they keep falling off? If your band is not tight enough and your shoulder straps keep falling off regardless of how high you adjust them, then you are wearing the wrong band size bra. Go down a size, and see if a more fitting band size gives you better support while keeping your shoulder straps in place. Now look at the cups of your bra. Do they fit and hold your breasts nicely, or do you see your breasts bulging and spilling out of the cup? If the latter is the case, choose a bigger cup that fits and supports you completely without bulging on the top, sides, or under your arms. When buying a new bra, try it with and without clothes to see how it shapes your breasts under the clothes. Well-fitted bras help you to keep your breasts looking perkier and to prevent them from sagging.

Here are other tips to help you look fabulous regardless of the style you choose:

Choose the right colors to accentuate your features and disguise other body parts: dark colors to slim and lighten and bright colors to add volume.

Use accessories to add a finishing touch to your outfit. Make sure they are subtle and not overwhelming.

Choose the right shoes. Shoes should be comfortable and appropriate for the occasion. You may match them to the color of your dress or to the color of your accessories. For instance, if you are wearing a black dress, you might accessorize with a white pearl necklace and white purse. Shoes could be black to match your dress or white to match your purse.

Choose your outfits to please the eye not to cause them to hurt. For instance, when wearing a striped or patterned blouse or a skirt, keep the rest of the outfit in solid colors.

Buy your accessories keeping your body shape and size in mind. For instance, while long dangling earrings and thick necklaces look great on a tall woman with a long neck, they might look overwhelming on a short and petite woman.

You can also browse fashion magazines. Many online stores such as Nordstrom, Macy's, and Bloomingdales now offer mix-and-match outfit suggestions with accessories included. Developing your own style might take a little time and practice, but keep in mind that a great outfit should be complimented by a charming personality. Yves Saint Laurent once said, "*What is important in a dress is the woman who is wearing it.*" Princess Diana and Grace Kelly are remembered not only for their great sense of style and elegance but also for their empathy, tact, grace, and humility.

YOUR FACE - A COVER OF WHO YOU ARE

Glowing Skin

Now let's talk about how to maintain and improve the health and appearance of your skin, which is the front page cover of who you are and is another important part of transforming your image. You can cover up and reshape your figure with the proper clothes, but your skin, especially on your face, is open for view most of the time and reflects your inner physical health. We discussed previously simple daily skin-care routines that will help to keep your skin looking younger and healthier longer. Now Ellen Gavrielov, a certified specialist in cosmeceuticals and fragrance production will teach us what ingredients to look for when buying cosmetic products and how to choose the right products appropriate for your skin type.

Choosing the Right Cosmetic Products

Currently the market trends in produce and skin care are increasingly becoming organic, GMO-free, and natural. Have you noticed? If you're going to make conscious decisions about what foods you'll be consuming, you should definitely make conscious decisions about the products you are applying to your skin. Why? Because the skin is the largest organ in our body and it absorbs 60% of what we put on it. So if you're applying products with toxins in them to your skin, you're making yourself toxic, yet your body will have a difficult time of ridding itself of these toxins. Eating healthy products is great for your skin says Ellen Gavrielov, but your skin should be fed healthy ingredients too. Products that claim to be organic or natural require a certificate to support these claims. Therefore, formulations must meet the COSMOS-standard and use only approved raw materials and certified ingredients that the Standard allows.

Visit a website www.cosmos-standard.org for more information about what the COSMOS-standard covers. *"COSMOS ORGANIC"* or *"COSMOS NATURAL"* will always appear right below the logo of the responsible certifier or association. Please visit the COSMOS website for definitions of these two certifications. The USDA is another organic certification stamp that may be found on labels. This organization has its own labeling guidelines and products must comply with USDA standards if they wish to carry the USDA Organic Seal. The three classifications based on the percentage of organic ingredients in the products are 100% organic, organic, and made with organic ingredients. For definitions and a list of USDA certified organic products, visit a website www.usdaorganicskincare.com.

Reading the ingredients label on cosmetic products is just as vital as reading the ingredients label on the packaged foods we buy. The concept in labeling is the same; the ingredients with the highest percentage are listed first and the lowest percentage last. It is important to read the labels carefully and choose your products accordingly. The best products to choose are those that contain natural extracts and herbal oils as there are many different types of plants that are beneficial for our skin. Products that contain a high concentration of high quality extracts will help maintain our skin health as well as improve certain skin conditions. The first rule of thumb is to avoid any facial product that contains mineral oil and petroleum as these will clog your pores (higher quality products will not use these cheap materials). Also, it's best to avoid detergent-based ingredients such as *sodium lauryl sulfate* or *sodium laureth sulfate* as these too are petroleum-based. Saponin-based surfactants are organically approved foaming alternatives to detergent surfactants. Saponin-containing plants you should look for in cosmetic cleansers include horse chestnut, licorice, soap bark, panama bark, soapwort, sarsaparilla, and yucca tree.

Here are some other ingredients Ellen Gavrielov recommends that you should avoid:

- Fragrances — Chemical fragrances in products are irritating and tend to dry out the skin. Opt for products that use essential oils or fruit and plant extracts to scent their solutions.
- Petroleum and mineral oil-derived ingredients such as propylene glycol, paraffin, mineral oil, butylene glycol, isopropyl alcohol, and petrolatum should be avoided.
- Preservatives such as formaldehyde, quaternium-15, and parabens, which include butylparaben, methylparaben, and propylparaben, should be avoided. Opt for plant-derived ingredients such as ethylhexylglycerin or phenoxyethanol.
- Alcohols such as isopropyl alcohol, SD alcohol 40, and ethyl alcohol erode the skin's barrier.

Ellen's Guide to Cosmetic Products

Normal Skin Type

Cleanse — Cleansing lotions that are water based are the best types of cleansers for this skin type. Look for plants such as cornflower, cleavers, blackberry, agrimony, bearberry, shinleaf, clary sage, strawberry, and honeysuckle.

Exfoliate — Both chemical and physical exfoliation methods are effective for this skin type; however, a combination of both will work synergistically.

Tone — The best toners to use are ones that are anti-aging as they are loaded with antioxidants, which are beneficial for normal skin types. These toners are formulated to keep your skin acting normally while defending against factors that lead to signs of aging.

Moisturize — Opt for a lightweight cleanser with anti-aging ingredients and the plants listed above.

Combination Skin Type

Look for extracts such as evening primrose, kukui, camellia, Roman chamomile, carrot, and tomato.

Cleanse — Since this skin type is a mixture of normal areas and an oily T-zone, the skin may react differently in different climates. Use a cleanser formulated for oily skin during the hot summer days and during the harsh winter, use a cleanser formulated for normal/dry skin.

Exfoliate — Exfoliate twice weekly with a gentle scrub. If you experience some breakouts, use a chemical exfoliant instead to avoid spreading bacteria from active lesions.

Tone — Look for a toner that contains an alcohol content of 4–15%. An alcohol agent will be listed in the middle to end of the ingredients label. Spritz the toner on your face (avoid spraying your eyes) after cleansing or exfoliating, and use a cotton pad to wipe your skin and remove excess dirt. This should be done once in the morning and once in the evening. If you suffer from breakouts, use an astringent such as witch hazel on the breakout areas, but avoid touching the drier parts of the skin.

Moisturize — Use a lightweight moisturizer that contains natural oils such as those listed above. Apply a pea-sized amount, and use your fingers to help spread the moisturizer around your skin, avoiding your eyes and the skin surrounding your eyes.

Dry Skin Type

Natural plant extracts used for this skin type are elderflower, aloe vera, orchid, mallow, St. John's wort, acacia, coltsfoot, quince, comfrey, and honey.

Cleanse — Look for cleansing creams that contain higher concentrations of oil, water, and emollients that soften the skin. Rose water, aloe vera, and glycerin are ingredients you should look for in your cleansers.

Exfoliate — Use a chemical exfoliator once a week and a facial scrub two times a week. Give your skin a couple of days between exfoliating.

Tone — Use a freshener that has zero alcohol content. Alcohol will further dry your skin, which is what we are trying to avoid. Look for the ingredients listed above.

Moisturize — Use a thicker cream with humectants such as propylene glycol and sorbitol to lock in moisture. Moisturize twice a day to help replenish moisture to your skin.

Oily Skin Type

Products for oily skin should contain extracts that have antibacterial properties such as tea tree oil, spiraea ulmaria extract, rosemary extract, cinnamon extract, and balm mint extract. Additionally, products for oily skin should contain components that will help regulate sebum such as nordihydroguaiaretic acid, niacinamide, yeast extract, horse chestnut extract, zinc gluconate, sarcosine and Enantia bark.

Look for products labeled "non-comedogenic", "non-acnegenic," and "oil-free."

Cleanse: — Look for a gentle foaming cleanser that contains deep penetrating ingredients such as the soapbark tree. Don't punish your skin with harsh cleansers; they can irritate your skin and cause the skin to produce more oil.

Exfoliate — You should exfoliate three times a week, allowing your skin to recuperate in between. A combination of chemical exfoliation and the use an abrasive tool like a facial sponge can be used once a week to help shed dead cells. Look for products containing salicylic acid, lactic acid, sulfur, papain, and pumpkin. As we previously discussed, these agents digest dead cells and help clear pores, which avoids impactions.

Tone — We are looking for a high degree of astringency from plants including witch hazel, lily, willow, dandelion, linden, and avens. The toner should also contain salicylic acid to exfoliate dead skin that can clog pores.

Moisturize — Always opt for an "oil-free" lotion, which is lighter than a cream. Look for oil- absorbing ingredients such as kaolin, bentonite, and diatomaceous earth. In the morning, you should apply and oil free moisturizer that contains an SPF, or you can apply an oil-free SPF on top of the moisturizer.

Sensitive Skin Type

Those with this skin type need to use products that deliver effective results to reduce redness and soothe irritation. Read the label, and look for ingredients that carry anti-inflammatory properties such as the calendula officinalis flower, azulene, red hogweed acetyl tetrapeptide-15, oat, vitamin E, ginger and bisabolol. The formulation should also contain agents that mimic the skin's natural composition of ceramides (substances that serve as part of the "glue" that holds surface skin cells together), which will fortify the skin's barrier and keep future irritants out. These agents include borage seed, evening primrose oil, avocado, sunflower, aloe vera, and comfrey. Avoid the following components that can cause stinging, burning, or facial redness: alcohol, witch hazel, menthol, peppermint, eucalyptus oil, clove oil, sulfates, fragrances, lactic acid, azelaic acid, benzoic acid, glycolic acid, vitamin C, AHAs, and parabens.

Cleanse — Look for "soap-free" and "oil free" on the label. It is best to use organic products for this skin type since you should avoid all the harsh chemicals and toxic ingredients that can be found in many cleansers. Cleanse morning and night.

Exfoliate — Abrasive tools and mechanical exfoliants are much too harsh for your skin type. It is best to use an enzyme-based chemical exfoliator once a week that is formulated for sensitive skin. If you find that this type of exfoliation is too harsh, you should try to make your own exfoliator with ingredients from your fridge!

Tone — Skin fresheners are formulated with 0–4% alcohol and therefore are the best options to tone this skin type. For a redness relief type of toner, look for one that contains the anti-inflammatory agents listed above.

Moisturize — Look for a moisturizer that is fragrance-free and contains the barrier-repairing properties listed above. Apply moisturizer twice a day: in the morning before makeup application and once in the evening before bed. Follow the application instructions on the product.

Chapter 15

TRANSFORMING YOUR HEALTH

"Take care of your body. It is the only place you have to live". Jim Rohn

Previous chapters discussed the importance and benefits of following a healthful, nutritious diet and incorporating regular exercise into your daily routine. Following a healthful lifestyle is an essential building block to overall balance and wellness. This chapter will focus on other steps you can take to prevent or detect and treat health problems in a timely manner. We will cover the most current thinking about having screening tests, recognizing different symptoms that you might be experiencing, and talking to your health care practitioner so you can get the best outcome from your visit.

Your Routine Checkups

Routine screening is age dependent and differs for every woman based on her medical and family history. For healthy women, ages 20–40, routine testing includes the following:

Dental Checkups — a routine cleaning is recommended to be done twice a year, or more often if needed, to check for gum disease and other oral problems.

Skin Exam — Annual skin assessments are recommended to be done, preferably by your health care provider, who knows what to look for. If you enjoy sunbathing, you might consider including a dermatologist on your wellness team. There are a few schools of thought regarding sun exposure. Some practitioners recommend avoiding the sun's rays between the hours of 10 a.m. and 2 p.m. and using sunscreen 100% of the time, while others encourage sunbathing any time of day without sunscreen. There is general agreement across the board that *sunburn* is to be avoided. The point here is that protection on some level is important. You should make the final decision regarding how to protect yourself by taking into consideration how fair your skin, hair, and eyes are. The rule of thumb is that those with light colored skin, hair, and eyes burn their skin much faster and may not be able to adequately depend on their own production of melanin than people with darker toned skin, hair, and eyes do. Discuss your thoughts, ideas, and concerns with your health care provider or dermatologist.

Eye Exam — It is a good idea to check your eyes, ideally when you are young, to establish a baseline, especially if you have a family history of eye problems such as glaucoma, cataracts, or macular degeneration. Documentation of your retina (retinal imaging) is very important, especially for people living with various health conditions including obesity, diabetes, high blood pressure, and issues with cholesterol. Retinal imaging refers to a photo taken of the back of the eye, which is NOT "invasive" since it is done by a machine that does not touch you directly. The retinal scan is performed by a trained optometrist or ophthalmologist. It involves dilating the pupil with drops so that a photo can be taken with a specialized camera. Your vision stays blurry after the exam for a few hours, so bringing a friend to drive you home might be an important consideration if your exam is scheduled during daylight hours. Read more about the value of retinal imaging here: www.vsp.com/retinal-exam.html

GYN Exam — A pelvic exam, Pap smear, and STD screening are tools used to make sure that early intervention addresses any issues before they become diseases. The recommendation by the CDC in 2014

was that women between the ages of 21–65 have routine annual exams to detect sexually transmitted infections such as HPV (human papillomavirus), which might cause cervical cancer. The reality is that even if a woman has one sexual partner, she is also exposing herself to every other sex partner that her one partner ever had. Discuss your relationship openly with your partner, and communicate as needed with your gynecologist so you can maintain optimal health.

Blood Test — As we discussed in previous chapters, the blood tests needed for each woman depend her symptoms, complaints, and family history, which will detect any predispositions. For relatively young and healthy women, common blood tests include a CBC (complete blood count), a chemistry and lipid profile to check for cholesterol and electrolytes, and a vitamin D level check, especially for those living in northern hemispheres where sun exposure is limited.

For women over 40, there are additional recommendations that, depending on the school of thought followed by you and your primary provider will affect your personal health decisions.

Mammogram — Exposure to x-rays, genetic predisposition, lifestyle, and what types of foods we consume (organic, processed etc.) are all considerations that affect how often you may wish to subject your breasts to this type of exam. The American Cancer Society recommends routine annual mammograms after the age of 40. Read more regarding the benefits and risks of annual mammography screening at www.cancer.org

Bone Density Scan — This screening is done to detect osteoporosis and is generally recommended during or after menopause. Two tests are popular: bone mineral density (BMD) and dual-energy x-ray absorptiometry (DEXA), the latter of which is generally reserved for women over 65 years of age as it is done with more radiation. Some women might have a higher risk if they have chronic medical conditions such as seizure disorder, endocrine imbalances, kidney and liver problems, rheumatoid arthritis, celiac disease, and inflammatory bowel disease. For these women, a bone scan might be recommended prior to menopause and appropriate treatment initiated as needed.

Colorectal Screening — A rectal digital exam and colonoscopy are recommended after the age of 50 to detect colon cancer and treat it if necessary. Do discuss the pros and cons with your provider.

Blood Tests — Additional blood tests for hormonal imbalances might be needed for women over 40 to detect premenopausal and perimenopausal changes. As discussed previously, the thyroid gland, ovaries, and adrenal glands are interconnected and influence each other. To accurately detect and diagnose any hormonal imbalance, all 3 glands should be checked and treated accordingly. Other blood tests recommended are fasting insulin and glucose levels, Hemoglobin A_1C to detect blood sugar dysregulation and a predisposition to diabetes.

Getting Ready for Your Health Care Visit

By this point, you have hopefully decided to find time for yourself. Perhaps you've already set aside the hours necessary to schedule that long overdue visit to your health care practitioner. As you are organize and gather information, you are empowering yourself to get the most out of your visit. Since chances your health care provider will see you only for a brief period of time, the more organized you are in presenting significant information, the better the outcome of your visit. You are the best resource for information on the history of your health. Here are some tips to facilitate your organization:

- Make a folder or file to store all your medical information in one place so it is easily accessible to you when needed. Some online platforms such as WebMD Health Manager, NoMoreClipboard, and Microsoft HealthVault offer free personal health records management systems, which allow you to compile, manage, and share all your health information. What information should you gather that would be relevant to your health care provider?

- It is important to have an accurate family history of medical diseases. Even though it is not a guarantee that you will have the same illnesses as your parents and grandparents, knowing your predisposition to certain chronic illnesses might help your health care provider to check for them and optimize your care to prevent or at least to decrease your chances of developing the same illnesses.

- Have a copy of your previous blood work, diagnostic results, and medical records from previous health care providers that you've visited. You have a right to obtain and keep copies of your test results and medical notes. Ask your health care practitioner to provide you with copies, and keep them for your own records.

- Make a list of all the medications, supplements, herbal remedies, and herbal teas that you are consuming with their respectful dosages and time taken during the day. Many supplements and herbal remedies can interact with prescription drugs; If possible, bring bottles of your medications and supplements with you to share with your health care provider.

Make a chronological spreadsheet of your symptoms progression. List the following information in the example below:

Symptoms	Started/ Stopped	Treatment	Treatment Results	Comments& Concerns
Example: Irregular spotting between periods	Started in 2007 after delivery of my son	Diagnosed: endometrial polyp. Removed in 2009 -started Birth Control pills	Symptoms stopped for 2 years; returned 6 months ago	Would like to consider alternative treatment to Birth Control pills

Communicating with Your Health Care Provider

Now that you are organized and have gathered all the necessary information, it is time to visit your health care provider. Communicating with your health care provider is one of the most important (as well as the most challenging) aspects of your visit. There are limits and time constrains for patient visits; most health care providers—even if willing—often do not have enough time to spend with each patient. Therefore, staying organized and being prepared for your visit will make a big difference in the outcome.

Dr. Ronald Hoffman, one of the nation's top experts on natural and alternative therapies and the medical director of the Hoffman Center in New York City, wrote an excellent book titled, *How to Talk with Your Doctor*. In his book, Dr. Hoffman provides detailed information for patients and health care practitioners about different medical conditions and their conventional and alternative treatment options. The information in the book is supported by an extensive resource list and reliable research sites. Dr. Hoffman's book offers suggestions for patients and health care providers on how to communicate more effectively as well as how to develop a stronger patient-doctor partnership. Below are some of the suggestions from Dr. Hoffman for effectively communicating with your health care provider:

- Bring a list or actual bottles of your prescriptions, over-the-counter medications, and supplements with you to the visit. (You may also photograph them with your mobile device and bring photos with you.) Explain why you are taking them, and report accurate dosages of your supplements and medications.

- Provide a list of all the health care practitioners, therapists, and alternative practitioners that you are seeing, and describe the types of treatments you are receiving from them.

- Discuss your diet and eating habits; ask for suggestions to improve them if necessary.

- Describe your symptoms accurately, and stay focused on the most important details pertinent to your health care problem.

- Don't hesitate to discuss your feelings and emotions, especially if you are feeling isolated and depressed.

- Be informed and proactive about your care, but leave the diagnosing of your problem to your health care practitioner. Self-diagnosing your illness by reading other people's blog's and Facebook posts is not the best way to deal with your medical problems. If you interested to review information about a particular symptom you are experiencing there are several reliable websites such as MyEllectronicMD.com and WebMD, which are symptom checkers that offer step-by-step instructions for evaluating your symptoms.

Here are some other things to remember when communicating with your health care provider:

- Be honest and speak up if you don't feel comfortable or do not understand the diagnosis or instructions provided.

- Bring a list of questions to ask your health care provider, and take notes during the visit. The information provided might sometimes be overwhelming, so ask for written instructions or bring another person with you for emotional support and to help you to understand the information provided.

- Discuss all the treatment options available for your diagnosis, including alternative treatments.

- Get detailed information on the benefits and side effects of particular treatments, what to expect, and how long will it take to see results.

You may also ask for suggestions on literature to read on any particular health topic. Being informed means staying proactive about your health and it is an important ingredient in a recipe to regain your energy, keep your symptoms under control, and live a healthy, full, and enjoyable life.

Chapter 16

TRANSFORMING YOUR FITNESS

"People with fitness goals succeed because they know where they are going."
Felicity Luckey

You finally signed up for a gym or bought equipment for your home gym, and you decided to start exercising. Congratulations! You checked with your health care provider, and were given permission to exercise, now what? Do you feel like you don't know where to start? Let's go over some basic information that you need to have before beginning your exercise regimen. If you are a beginner, or haven't exercised for a long time, your goal is to choose an exercise regimen in order to establish a basic level of fitness. This means you want to target all areas, in general, to improve your overall function. A sample exercise routine would include a cardio workout, flexibility, strength, stabilization, and core. This focuses on your functional conditioning and cardiovascular endurance. Once you feel stronger and comfortable with your routine, your level of fitness may progress to more complex exercises. You might ask, "For how long and how often should I exercise?" Answers to these questions depend on your level of fitness, the goals you are trying to achieve, and the type of exercises you are performing. For instance, the recommendation for stretches and core exercises is to perform these daily. Weight training and cardio workouts work best when done at intervals with one or two days of rest in between. Also it is important to pay attention to your body reaction to exercises. That is, if you feel mildly tired but mostly energized after a workout, this would be a good sign, and it suggests that you should continue at the same level. If you feel more tired and exhausted after exercising, this might indicate that you are doing too much and may need to decrease the intensity of your exercise regimen. As discussed previously, people with adrenal and chronic fatigue are not able to tolerate intense exercise routines. If this is your case, it is best to begin with a 20-minute daily walk, until treatment for your condition resolves your symptoms. As you feel better you may slowly increase the intensity of your workout as tolerated. Marcin Machula, PES recommends following these basic rules when exercising to avoid injuries and obtain the greatest benefits from your routine:

Stretches – Daily performance is optimal. Muscles need to be warmed up before stretching to avoid injury; preferably performed after cardio or weightlifting exercises.

Strength training – Select proper weight for your routine to avoid injury. For beginners start with light weights (2-5 lbs) and progress as tolerated. Organize your exercises in repetitions and sets, with rest periods in between. For instance, a sample exercise could be 10-12 repetitions per set with 30-60 seconds of rest between sets.

Core training is best if performed everyday with 10-15 repetitions per set. Important to breath properly by inhaling during muscle relaxation and exhaling during muscle contraction.

Cardiovascular training, for beginners, should start with gentle exercise such as walking, increasing gradually as your body tolerates. Try to alternate your cardio routine with different forms of exercises to engage different muscle groups in your body.

Drink water before and during your exercise routine. This helps to replenish fluids in your tissues and muscles

Do not exercise if you have a fever, high blood pressure, chest pain, extreme fatigue, dizziness, low blood pressure, bleeding, and muscle pain or injury.

Choose appropriate clothes and shoes for your cardio workout. Buy a pair of comfortable walking shoes which have a good cushioning in the insole and support your ankles.

MARCIN'S GUIDE TO OFFICE/HOME FITNESS

Now that we are done with the basic guidelines, it is time to go over the fitness program itself. This program is easy to follow - even for beginners, and may be performed anywhere, including your office at work, home gym, or in the hotel while you travel. It doesn't require any equipment besides your own body and a set of light weights (i.e. dumbbells or bottles of water for arm strengthening). The program consists of 4 parts which include core training, stretching, weight training and a cardiovascular workout. So let's get started.

WARM UPS

It is important to warm-up appropriately before starting any exercise regimen. Warming up prevents injury to your muscles and joints, improves your mobility and prepares your body for the exercises at hand. Warm-up exercises are simple to do and don't take a long time. You could start with simple movements such as hip circles, torso circles, leg swings and high knee march. You could also include the following exercises listed below: jumping jacks, torso twist and body weight squats. This warm-up routine takes only 5 minutes to complete; each exercise is 30-60 seconds long.

1. Jumping Jacks

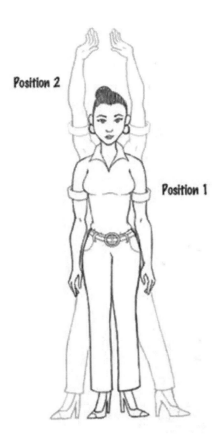

- Stand with your feet close, arms extended, along your body
- At the same time clap your hands over your head and jump your feet out to the sides.
- Jump back and reverse it to the starting position.
- Repeat 10-20 times.
- Insert image

2. Torso Twists

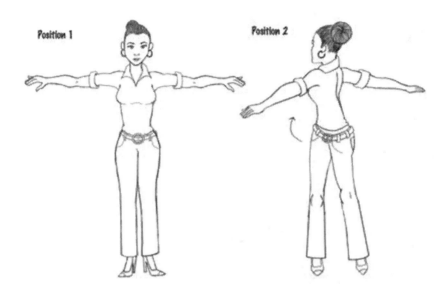

- Stand with your feet shoulder width apart
- Bring your extended arms to your shoulder level
- Keeping your abs tight rotate your upper body from side to side, making sure that your arms stay up throughout the whole set.
- Repeat 10-20 times.

3. Body Weight Squat.

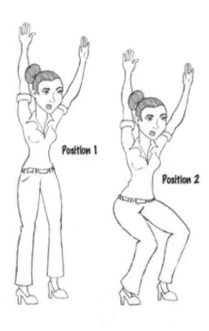

- Stand with your feet shoulder-width apart, toes pointing forward and knees over your toes. Keep your hands raised up over your head.
- Contract your abdominal muscles. Slowly begin to squat down, bending knees and flexing hips, keeping feet straight (as if sitting into a chair). Don't allow any internal rotation at the hips or knees.
- Allow the pelvis to sit back while maintaining a neutral position of the spine.
- Put pressure through the heels to push up and return to starting position.
- Repeat 10-20 times

CORE EXERCISES

Core exercises are most beneficial when performed every day. At the beginner's level start with 10-12 repetitions- one set for each exercise. Increase gradually as tolerated to 15-20 repetitions per set, and workup to 2 sets.

1. Torso Twist

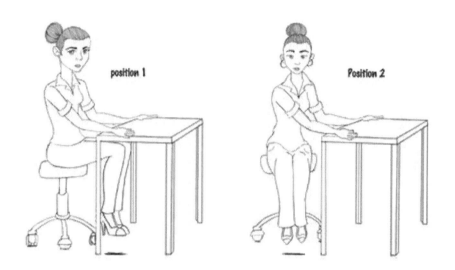

- Find a swivel chair. Sit upright with knees together and feet just off the floor.
- Hold the edge of the desk and, while engaging your core, use the chair to swivel from side to side.
- Go back and forth 10-12 times.

2. Squat With Offset

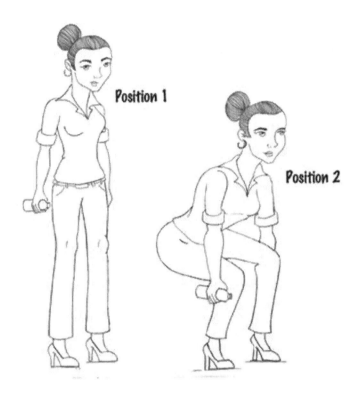

Position 1

Position 2

- Stand with your feet shoulder-width apart, head up, your back straight. Hold a weight in each hand.

- Keeping your body upright, contract your abdominal muscles, bend your knees and gradually lower yourself into a squat position until your thighs are parallel to the floor.

- Do not let your back round, and keep your knees tracking over your toes.

- Pause for 2 seconds and use your heels to raise into the starting position. Inhale on the way down and exhale on the way up.

- Repeat 10-12 times.

3. Wood Chop

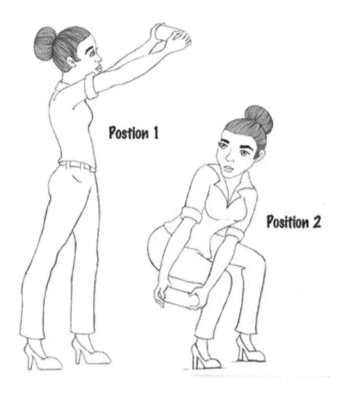

Postion 1

Position 2

- Stand up straight holding a weight with both hands.
- Keeping the arms straight, swing the weight in a controlled motion up across your left shoulder.
- Swing it back toward your right hip as you bend your knees into a squat position.
- Continue this chopping movement for 10-12 reps then switch sides.

4. Seated Leg Raises

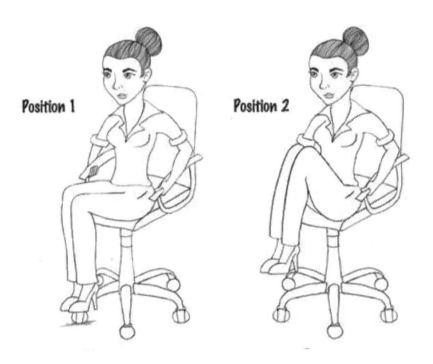

- Choose a chair with sturdy arms for this exercise.
- Sit up with your back straight and support your body with your forearms on the arms of the chair. Keep your legs straight.
- Breathe out as you raise your knees up and in to your chest, while rounding your lower back slightly
- Bring your weight off the chair and on to your forearms.
- Breath in and Slowly Lower your legs down straight
- Repeat 10-12 times

5. Torso Twist

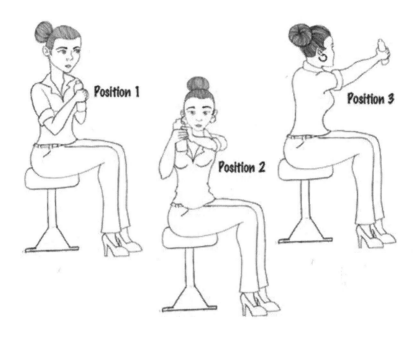

- Sit with your back straight and facing to the front. Hold a weight in both hands with your arms extended out in front at shoulder level.
- Contract abdominal muscles and twist your body to one side, turning your head, shoulders and hips and moving your feet.
- Twist back to the opposite side, while moving your hips and feet. Repeat 10- 12 times in each direction

STRENGTH EXERCISES

Strength training is not as complicated as it sounds and has great benefits such as developing muscles mass and decreasing body fat, if done properly. It includes slow controlled movements against some resistance, which could be your own body weight, lifting weights or resistance bands. Choosing an appropriate weight will depend on your level of fitness; for beginners start with light weights 1-3 lbs, and increase slowly and gradually as tolerated. Your muscles should feel slightly fatigued at the end of 10-12 reps with appropriate weights. Your muscles should feel slightly fatigued at the end of 10-12 reps with appropriate weights. As you get stronger and your reps become too easy to accomplish, increase weights gradually performing exercises very slowly and with control. Count to ten to help you to control your movements as you getting to desired position. Try to maintain tension in your muscles throughout the whole set of exercises; count to ten holding the position and to return to resting position.

1. Reverse Lunges.

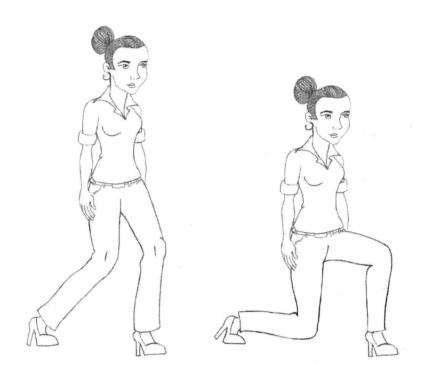

- Begin with both feet shoulder-width apart and pointed straight ahead.
- Place your hands on your hips and contract abdominal muscles
- Lunge backwards landing on the ball of your foot .Both knees should now be bent at 90 -degree angles, front foot should be flat on the ground and the back foot should have the heel lifted off the ground.
- From this position drive off back foot onto your front foot.
- Stand up to a balanced position on both legs. Repeat 10-12 times and switch to the other leg.

2. Warrior Squat

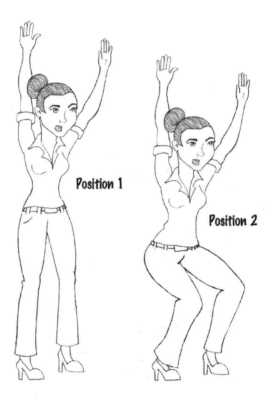

Position 1

Position 2

- Stand with your feet shoulder-width apart, toes pointing forward and knees over your toes. Keep your hands raised up over your head.

- Contract your abdominal muscles. Slowly begin to squat down, bending knees and flexing hips, keeping feet straight (as if sitting into a chair). Don't allow any internal rotation at the hips or knees.

- Allow the pelvis to sit back while maintaining a neutral position of the spine.

- Put pressure through the heels to push up and return to starting position.

- Repeat 10-12 times.

3. Cross Over Lunges

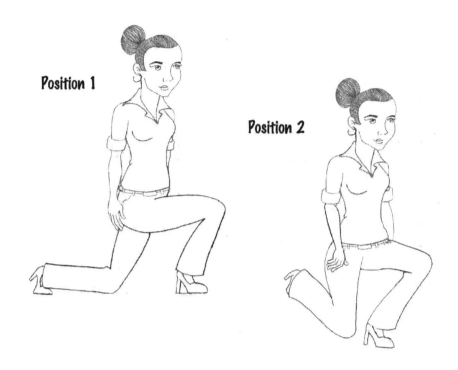

Position 1

Position 2

- Begin with both feet shoulder-width apart and pointed straight ahead.
- Place your hands on your hips and contract abdominal muscles
- Step forward and across in front of your other leg
- Lower your body down, keeping your head up and upper body upright.
- Stand up to a balanced position on both legs.
- Repeat 10-12 times and switch to the other leg.

4. Incline Push Up

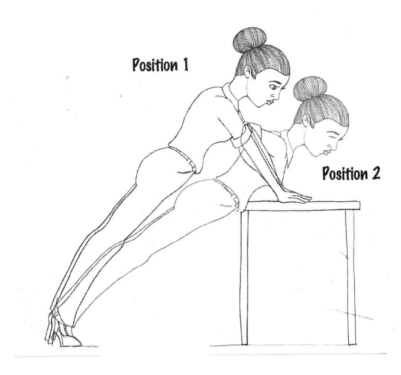

- Position yourself in a push up position, facing a sturdy desk or it can be a wall.
- Keep your feet shoulder-width apart
- Keep your hands on a desk/wall wider than shoulder width
- Keep your body straight from head to toe and contract your abdominal muscles
- Slowly bend your arms and lower your body, maintain the tension in your muscles, and hold the position for 20- 30 seconds
- Exhale and return to starting position.
- Repeat 10-12 times.

5. Bent Over Row

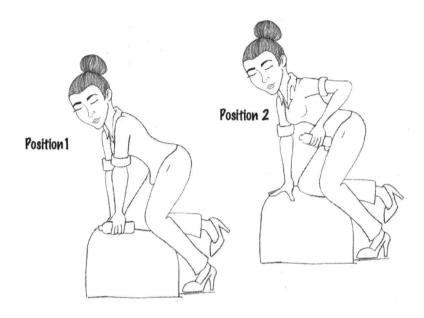

- Kneel on a bench/chair holding a weight in one hand and supporting your body with the other arm
- Keep your back flat and contract your abdominal muscles
- Bend your elbow and lift the dumbbell up to the side of your chest
- Pause for a second and lower the dumbbell back, returning to a starting position
- Repeat 10-12 times and switch to the other side.

FLEXIBILITY EXERCISES

Stretches are an important part of any exercise regimen and are recommended to be done on daily basis. Stretches need to be performed when your muscles are warmed up, since stretching cold muscles could cause injury and pain. It is best when stretches are performed after cardio or strength training routine. If you are not doing a vigorous exercise routine that day, do at least simple warm up exercises as mentioned above, before stretching your muscles. Hold each stretch 10-30 seconds and repeat 3-5 times.

1 Calves

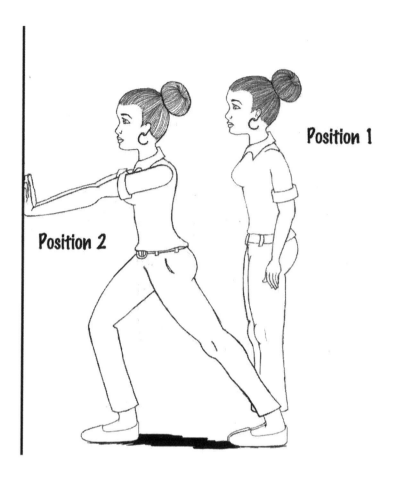

Position 1

Position 2

- Stand facing a wall and place your hands in front of you.
- Bend one leg forward toward the wall for support and keep the other leg straight behind you about 3 feet
- Lean against the wall and stop movement when slight tension is felt.
- Hold for 10-30 sec; switch sides and repeat on each leg 3-5 times

2   Hamstring

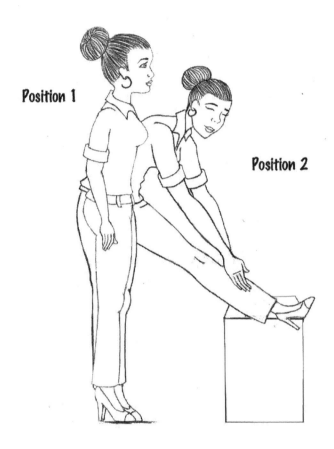

Position 1

Position 2

- Stand straight with one leg propped up on a chair or bench in front of you.
- Keep the propped leg straight and
- Slightly lean forward at the hip until you feel a slight stretch in the back of your legs.
- Hold for 10-30 sec; Switch sides and repeat on each leg 3-5 times

3   Quads

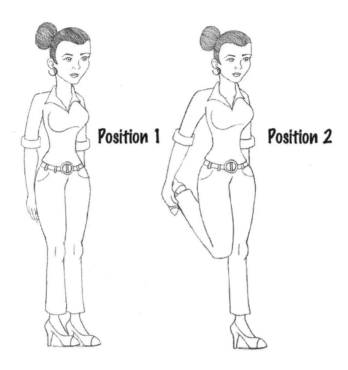

Position 1   Position 2

- Stand with your feet shoulder-width apart,
- To maintain a balance you may place your hand on a wall or hold the back of the chair
- Bend one foot behind you by flexing your knee.
- Hold your foot and slowly bring it closer to your buttock until you feel tension in your thigh
- Hold for 10-30 sec, Switch sides and repeat on each leg 3-5 times

4   Seated Back Stretch

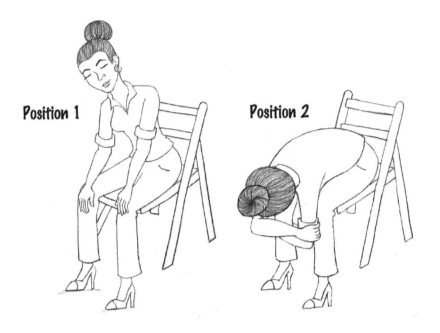

Position 1

Position 2

- Seat on a chair and spread your feet apart
- From the seated position, gently lean your torso forward with your arms until you start feeling a gentle tension in your upper and lower back
- Hold this position for 10 -30 seconds. Repeat 3 - 5 times.

5 Seated Reach

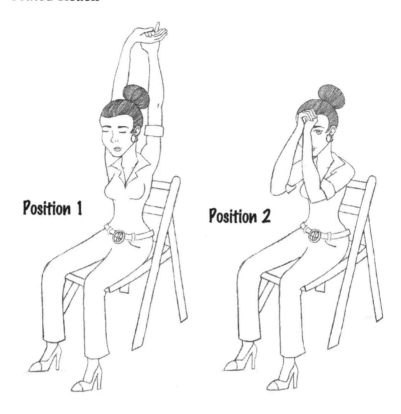

- Seat upright on a chair and spread your feet apart
- From the seated position, gently bring your arms straight overhead
- Your shoulders should go towards your ears.
- Stretch until you start feeling a gentle tension in your upper arms
- Hold this position for 10 -30 seconds. Repeat 3 - 5 times.

6   Seated Back Twist

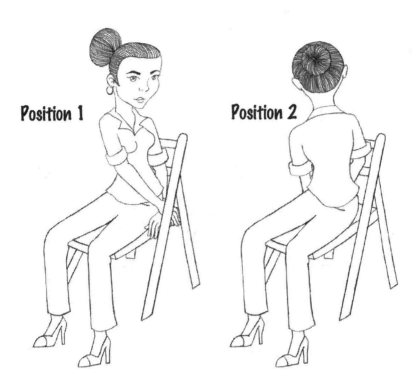

- Seat upright on a chair and spread your feet apart
- From the seated position, gently turn your head and shoulders to the right side
- Twist your torso and place your hands at the side of the chair
- Hold for 10-30 sec, Switch sides and repeat 3-5 times

CARDIO-VASCULAR EXERCISES

Cardio workouts are a definite plus to any routine; however, if you are a beginner or haven't exercised for a long time, it might be challenging to engage in it. As was previously discussed, cardiovascular exercises benefit your overall health. This is described in greater detail, and with additional points regarding different types of exercises on pages .... This section of the book will address how to start and how to safely and appropriately perform your cardio workout. For beginners, it is recommended that you start with simple walking and counting steps. It is relatively safe for anyone, simple to follow, and may be done anywhere. All that is required is a pair of good, supportive walking shoes. Just to be clear, we are talking about brisk walking - not a leisure stroll in the park. For walking to be effective and to have cardio benefits, you would need to raise your heart rate up. Other alternatives to walking would be stair climbing or cycling, which are a bit more advanced. Start your walking routine slowly for about 20-30 minutes per day, target counting your steps (you could buy a pedometer to help you), and aim for 60,000-100,000 steps per week as a beginner. Count steps every day and throughout the day. As you get stronger, you might advance your cardio workout by increasing the intensity and the lengths of your exercise routine.

I know as a busy woman myself, finding a specific time for cardio workout could be a challenging endeavor. An excellent alternative is following a 'bursting' style fitness workout. It includes varying degrees of intensity in 15-20 minutes workouts, which could be broken down and performed at 5-minute intervals throughout the day. It might be a bit intense for a beginner, so try it out and see how your body responds. The basic idea is to alternate intensity of your exercise between short periods. For instance, if you are walking, then alternate short periods (1 -3 minutes, as tolerated) of brisk walking with sprinting or jogging. You could also use a jump rope and alternate it with high knee marching, or use stairs to climb up fast and down slowly. You could also use a portable stepping machine. It is relatively small in size and could be kept in the office if needed. Remember to warm-up first, before doing any exercise, in order to avoid injury. Other alternatives for advanced aerobic activity: you might invest in a DVD led aerobic workout or, if time permits, sign up for cardio workout classes in the gym. Regardless of the type of activity you choose and prefer, your main goal is to do it consistently. As a beginner always start slow, and progress gradually as your body adapts to your routine. Because every woman is different, there is no single exercise routine that will work for everybody. You are welcome to use information in this book and suggested beginners level exercises listed to incorporate in your routine.

Add exercises to you daily calendar; remember, you don't have to perform all the exercises at once. Weight training and cardio workout are recommended to be done 3 times a week, and core and stretching - if possible, on a daily basis. You could spread them out through the day and alternate days of weight training and cardio workouts. The most important thing would be to listen to your body. Treat yourself with love, and don't push too hard if your body is feeling tired and exhausted. Give yourself time to adjust and change. With these points in mind you should find yourself well along your road to healing and transformation

Chapter 17

TRANSFORMING YOUR DIET

"The food you eat can be either the safest and most powerful form of medicine or the slowest form of poison." Ann Wigmore

Have you ever tried to change your diet? Have you moved from one diet to another only to discover that following rules became so confusing or complex that you gave up trying to follow them altogether? If so, you might have quit out of frustration, anger, or dissatisfaction because your goals were not met.

Here's the good news: If you are ready to revamp your diet once and for all, this part of the book is for you. I will now focus on changing your eating habits, which can help you to learn how to enrich your daily diet with the very best nourishing, balanced, and satisfying meals. Rather than spending energy on losing weight or trying a diet for a few weeks only to fail and give up, we will concentrate on taking one step at a time towards healthier meal planning. This method helps you succeed and celebrate small accomplishments, get your family and children on board, and transform you and your relationship with food.

Previously, we discussed how to clean your kitchen and your environment. By now, I hope you have or are planning to purchase safe and healthy kitchenware and cookware as well as a quality water filtering system for your house or for your kitchen. I hope you did your research and know which foods are safe and healthy to eat and which foods need to be avoided. The next step is taking an inventory of your kitchen cabinets and lists the products that you use to cook your food and feed your family.

Here is the list of Dos and Don'ts for your healthy eating plan:

SUGARS

Do use alternatives such as raw honey, stevia, maple sugar, brown rice syrup, agave nectar, Sucanat, and coconut sugars sparingly as needed.

Don't include products containing refined sugars, artificial sweeteners, or high fructose corn syrup in your diet

FATS

Do use small amounts of organic butter and vegetable oil such as olive oil, grapeseed oil, and avocado oil.

Don't consume products that contain high amounts of saturated fats or hydrogenated vegetable oils, such as margarine or shortenings. Try to avoid processed and refined oils, such as corn oil, sunflower oil, canola oil, cottonseed oil, safflower and soybean oil.

PROTEINS

Do add a variety of high-protein containing foods to your meals; choose healthier proteins from plants, fish, nuts, legumes, poultry, and lean cuts of meats

Don't eat proteins from processed meats such as hot dogs, bacon, cold cuts, and sausages. They are high in saturated fat and sodium and have tons of other chemicals used as preservatives.

CAFFEINE

Do switch to a healthier alternative such as water processed decaf coffee, or drink tea instead. Black and green tea do contain caffeine but in smaller amounts; green tea is rich in antioxidants

Don't drink caffeinated beverages such as soda or energy drinks. (Taper off rather than abruptly stop drinking coffee; do this by decreasing consumption gradually over time to prevent withdrawal.) As we discussed previously, coffee is a strong stimulant and will drain your adrenal glands. Decrease consumption to avoid adrenal fatigue.

ALCOHOL

Do drink small amounts of red wine—no more than 1 glass (4 ounces) a day—if approved by your health care provider.

Don't drink alcohol regularly. There is enough evidence to prove that regular drinking of alcohol containing products in large amounts could cause serious diseases such as liver problems, cancer, and birth defects if taken during pregnancy.

Simple Guide to Healthier Eating

Choose fresh foods in their most natural form; for example, choose eating a fresh apple over drinking concentrated apple juice.

Avoid processed, packaged foods when preparing your meals; try to use fresh and single ingredient food products to cook from scratch.

Start your day with a breakfast that includes protein, a healthy fat, and fiber.

Include a midmorning and mid-afternoon snack to avoid a feeling drop in energy and having food cravings.

Include fresh salads and vegetables to your meals—make these fill at least half of your plate.

Drink plenty of water throughout the day to keep your body well hydrated.

Add a variety of nuts to your daily food intake; you can have small amounts of raw nuts as a snack or add nut butters to your smoothies or as dips for your fruits and vegetables.

Eat non-fried fish several times a week. Use healthier varieties, which are wild caught and free of mercury and hormones.

Become a label reader. Look out for hidden fats, simple and artificial sugars, artificial colors and flavors, and any chemicals and ingredients used as preservatives.

Keep junk food out of your house and substitute it with healthier alternatives.

Learn to cook healthy meals at home, or be conscious when eating out (more details to follow).

Make healthy substitutions in your favorite recipes to enjoy your favorite foods.

PUTTING IT ALL TOGETHER

Now that we've covered some basics, it is time to roll up your sleeves and implement these changes into your daily life. Yes, I know that you are busy with endless tasks and responsibilities, and you are probably thinking, "The last thing I want to do is worry about my nutrition!" **Good news**! This part of the book offers easy-to-follow, step-by-step guidelines to help you implement these changes throughout your daily life. So let's get started.

Food Journal

The first step is to fill out a food diary. I recommend doing this for a week to see what your nutritional patterns and habits are. Although tedious, this process is essential. A food diary will help you to become more aware of the food choices you make on a daily basis. It is a good tool to assist you in assessing your nutritional deficits and may help you to implement necessary changes.

Your food diary should include at least 4 columns: (1) Time, (2) Food/drink consumed and its detailed description (how it was cooked, and what seasoning was added, etc.) (3) Portion—size or amount, (4) Notes—your reaction (energy, mood) to the food consumed. Here is a sample below:

Meal type	Time	Food/drink description	Portions/Amount	Comments
Breakfast	7:30 am	Scrambled eggs with spinach and tomatoes, green tea	2 eggs with vegetables and olive oil 8 oz cup of tea	Was groggy and not hungry in the morning
Morning snack	10:30 am	Apple with almond butter, water	1 medium size apple, 3 tbsp of butter	Was jittery and shaking before my snack

Be specific when you write comments and reactions to food eaten. Include how you felt (bloated, satisfied, rapid pulse, or sleepy) after eating a certain food. This helps you target any food sensitivities you might have. Follow your reactions as you selectively eliminate these foods.

In the "portion and amount" column, write the portion size of the food ingested. You might add the calorie content of the food if you like. There are various schools of thought regarding calorie counting. Some dieticians and nutritionists follow the rule that a certain amount of calories eaten equals a pound of body weight, while others pay more attention to the *type* of caloric intake (fat/ carb/ protein) and balance these in accordance with the body type of the individual seeking guidance. The assumption in this book is that we are all unique, and calorie intake is different for each individual since it is based on body type, metabolism, genetics, activity level, and personal health. In addition, women's caloric needs might differ depending on the time of the month, their metabolism, and their age. Each body requires varying amounts of nutrients depending on menstruation (we need more nutrients) and during menopausal years (when we require less calories and different nutrients). This chapter focuses on the value of the nutrition of the food; that is, the nutritional value is more significant than the number of calories a food provides. For example, a simple 3-inch glazed donut may have 260 calories, with 14 grams of fat (6 grams are saturated fats), 31 grams of carbs (12 grams of simple sugar), 3 grams of protein, 330 mg of sodium, and no vitamins or minerals whatsoever. When we compare these 260 "empty calories" to approximately 300 nutritional calories provided by a cup of oatmeal with raisins, dates, nuts, apples, blueberries, cinnamon, and milk (recipe provided later), we realize that this second choice of 260–300 calories is rich in fiber, healthy fats, and a list of vitamins and minerals. While you are welcome to count your calories, keep in mind that the nutritional value of your food choices remains the most important thing. A good tool for calorie counting is a free website www.CalorieKing.com, or you can use a super tracker at the USDA website: www.ChooseMyPlate.gov.

Once you have completed your food diary, look it over, and see if you notice any patterns. Check the foods you ate and your reactions, and see what you might be able to reduce, avoid, or replace. Are there healthful substitutions that you might consider for the next 7-day food diary?

Identify strategies to change and improve your nutrition. You don't need to try to do everything at the same time. The goal is to make changes slowly rather than overwhelm yourself. Develop a step-by-step plan of action. First, review your diary for healthful choices you have been making, mindfully or naturally. Consider tweaking a few meals to increase their health benefits. Choose 2–3 of the easiest and least time-consuming steps, and implement them slowly into your daily routine. Then, observe your reaction to these changes. Modify them if necessary. The easiest approach for me was to begin with healthy snacks (recipes to follow). This improvement took minimum preparation and was easy to implement as well as to monitor its progress. Do this for a week, a month, or for as long as needed until it becomes a habit. Then move on to the next step. There is no right or wrong way to do it. Choose whatever works best for you and your busy life.

TO COOK OR NOT TO COOK

Cooking doesn't have to be a rocket science. While, to some, cooking may represent a career and creatively artistic experience, to others it may be as simple as two steps: preparation time and cooking time. Unless you are interested in preparing elaborate dishes to be served in a French or Italian restaurant or are perhaps catering an extravagant affair, you will want to focus on cooking for yourself and your family with the goal being to simply prepare healthful and nutritious meals.

If you are as lucky as I am and already know how to cook, that's great. All you need to do is fine-tune your skills and learn how to tweak cooking methods i.e. from frying to baking/ steaming/broiling and from using rich salty or fatty sauces to learning how to flavorfully enhance foods with healthful herbs and spices.

If cooking has never been your favorite pastime, or if you feel uncomfortable with your lack of expertise, now is the perfect time to add a few simple skills to your list of talents. It is never too late to learn. With some time, patience, and practice, your previous experiences with burned or over-salted dishes will transform into healthfully delicious home-cooked meals you will be proud to serve. When cooking in your own home, you can control the quality of all ingredients as well as the type of preparation and portion size for you and your family.

I know you are probably saying right now, "I am too busy and don't have time to cook at home." This chapter offers makeover and substitution recipes to enhance your favorite meals as well as easy-to-make recipes that require minimal effort and little preparation time. If interested, please read on. If, however, you really do not have the opportunity to cook at home, or you eat out often due to your schedule, here are a few helpful suggestions to make your eating out experience more healthful:

Do your research, and locate restaurants in your area that offer organic and healthful foods.

Check restaurant menus online before eating out if possible to see what is being offered.

Consider drinking 8 ounces of pure water or eating a small healthful snack before you leave for the restaurant to avoid a ravenous appetite. This helps you resist the extra bread and appetizers offered.

Speak up and be ready to ask questions about the menu options; feel free to request vegetable substitutes for breads and pasta side dishes.

Choose first from the salad section, and eat some fresh greens and vegetables prior to the main entrée.

Avoid ordering fried food; choose steamed, sautéed, broiled, or baked vegetables, fish, poultry, and meat.

Choose lean varieties of your meat (i.e. sirloin) to avoid extra saturated fats in your meal.

Choose healthful grains and vegetables as side dishes; request brown instead of white rice, and yams over white potatoes (baked or fried).

Organize your plate when ordering a meal, and divide it in three parts: one part for your proteins (meat, poultry, or fish) should be the size of your palm or your iPhone; the second part for your grains/carbs should be the size of your fist or a tennis ball; fill the rest of your plate with salad and vegetables.

Limit your intake of appetizers, especially if fried or high in saturated fat.

Pay attention to how much alcohol you are consuming as alcohol is often high in calories and mixed drinks have high sugar content. It is easier to control the amount consumed when you sip slowly rather than drink quickly.

Choose your beverages wisely; avoid sodas and juices. While they may taste great, they have too much sugar or artificial sweeteners. Stick to plain flavored water or order teas instead.

Bring your own sauces and salad dressings since they are often prepared with bad oils, sugar, or Trans fats and might contain gluten. If possible ask for a separate olive oil and vinegar dressing.

Permit yourself an occasional treat, and enjoy it. Remember that your diet should be healthful most of the time; it is up to you to decide how often you wish to choose healthful/unhealthful foods. One day, it may be 90/10 or 80/20. Another day, you might just satisfy cravings. Try to aim to make healthful choices 80–90% of the time on a daily basis, leaving your 10–20 "less healthful choices" to occasional treats.

Getting Your Family On Board

The most challenging endeavor for me was to get my family—my kids and my husband—on board with healthful eating. Even though body weight was never an issue in my family, our diet did include fried foods, unhealthful fats, high fructose sweets, and other junk foods that are best avoided. At the beginning, the goal of getting my kids to start eating more fruits and vegetables seemed unattainable. Eventually, there was some progress—but the work is still ongoing.

The first step I took was to eliminate all the junk food from my house, which included leaving the following off my next grocery-shopping list: chips, cookies, sodas, juices from concentrates, candy, and sweets with artificial colors and flavors.

The second step was to stock my kitchen cabinets and refrigerator with a wide variety of fresh fruits and vegetables as well as more healthful versions of snacks. Since we don't have nut allergies, these snacks included nuts and dry fruits.

During the first week, I left a bowl of fresh fruits and some nuts and dry fruits on the table. When my kids wanted a snack after school or between meals, these foods were the only options available. They were easily accessible, and even though during that first week, the bowl of fruits was left untouched, as time progressed, the fruits became a regular part of our diet. What is more, when my kids have their friends over, they are also eating fruits now. Do my kids still eat chips and other junk food at school? Probably, yes, and I am okay with it. My goal was and is to educate my family without becoming a nag, being pushy, or coming across as a distraction to healthful choices. Over time, my family is adapting to and enjoying healthy living on a daily basis 80–90% of the time. Of course, we indulge during the other 10–20%—and this is allowed.

At the beginning, I also offered my family transition foods. These were more healthy versions of junk food. I substituted baked chips in lieu of fried chips. I purchased organic sodas. To me, chips and sodas are junk foods regardless of whether they are fried, baked, or organic. They might still be processed with preservatives. Kids would be better off eating fresh fruits and vegetables and avoiding processed foods completely. Below are other suggestions for helping your family transition to more healthful eating habits:

Don't be too restrictive. "Forbidden fruit," as we well know, is sweeter. The more you restrict the more resistance you might receive. Implement changes gradually, and allow for the occasional treat. Focus on what they can have.

Educate your family by explaining the benefit of healthful food choices. Make it understandable—use terms that kids understand and relate to.

Add nutritious foods like vegetables and legumes to food recipes if you need to mask their presence. For instance, my meatballs and meatloaf are only 50% meat, and the rest are vegetables. My family enjoys the flavor with or without a conversation about the ingredients.

Offer new foods to your family on a regular basis. Don't get discouraged if they don't embrace the newness on the first try. It might take some time to retrain their taste buds, so do persist.

Take your kids grocery shopping with you so they can be involved in the choices of foods as well as the preparation and cooking process. Kids are usually more willing to eat food that they prepared themselves.

Making smoothies and juices is another way to include vegetables and fruits in your kids' diets. Even bitter greens can be camouflaged in a well-balanced smoothie if combined with fruits and berries.

Use your creativity. For smaller kids, make food fun; arrange it in different shapes on their plate.

Bake and prepare healthful treats, substituting whole grain (or almond or coconut flour) for bleached flour. Avoid simple sugars and Trans fats, choosing more healthful alternatives.

KITCHEN BASICS 101

Hopefully by now you are encouraged enough to use your kitchen and cook for your family if not on daily basis, then at least several times during the week. Before diving into a list of recipes, let's first transform your kitchen to make it easier for you to cook quick and healthful recipes.

We've already discussed the importance of obtaining a water filter, throwing out your nonstick pots and pans, and using glass or BPA-free storage containers. Other kitchen basics include the following items:

- A set of 3–5 nesting bowls, which provide variety in size. They can be glass, enamel, or stainless steel and are used for mixing and food preparation.

- A set of pots and pans can be cast iron (these are heavy to lift) with or without ceramic coating (if they don't have ceramic coating, they need to be "seasoned," which you can look up online). Another option for pots and pans is stainless steel. The numbers and sizes you need of these depend on the size of your family.

- A slow cooker is one of my big helpers in the kitchen. It is useful in preparing dishes over a long period of time. Cooking one-dish meals in this appliance saves time in preparation and cleanup since multiple pots and pans are not needed.

- A pressure cooker is very helpful for cooking foods at a faster rate.

- A rice cooker helps to batch cook your grains with minimal effort. Just add grains and water; the cooker does the rest.

- A juicer is a good investment and helps add nutrients from fruits and vegetables to your diet.

- A high speed blender is great for making smoothies and soups. There are different varieties with varying sizes and speed levels. Examples include Vitamix, NutriBullet, and a few others that promise to make nutrients more bioavailable by mechanically breaking them down for easier digestion. Each of these has its plusses and minuses; do your research, and choose what is best for you and your family.

- A steamer is an excellent tool used to steam vegetables and to cook dumplings. There are metal and wooden varieties. Some sit on top of pots, while others nest within pots.

- A cutting board is a necessary tool. There are pros and cons to plastic, wood, ceramic, and other materials. Do your research to see what works best for you. Have at least one for meats and one for fruits and vegetables. Keep them separate, and wash them according to the manufacturers' guidelines before and after each use.

- A Food Saver vacuum sealing system is not a necessity but may be a good investment if you enjoy bulk cooking and freezing your meals.

- A chopper, grater, and slicer are "must-have" tools for any kitchen. Again, do your research and take into consideration your family size and the amount of cooking you will do in your kitchen when making you choices. Additionally, depending on your needs, you might consider investing in a food processor that performs several operations.

- Utensils for every kitchen include wooden utensils, which can be used with ceramic, cast iron, and stainless steel pots and pans.

- Other kitchen basics include a mixer, vegetable peeler and corer, garlic press, potato masher, baking sheets and pans, whisks, oven/stove-safe mitts, measuring cups and spoons, paper towels, and anything else that you personally want to have in your kitchen.

Now that you stocked your kitchen with basic equipment, it is time to stock your pantry with healthful and delicious foods.

Time Saving Cooking Tips For a Busy Woman

Start planning your meals ahead of time. The best way to do this is with a weekly schedule; set weekly menus, and do grocery shopping a week ahead.

Consider your schedule for the coming week to plan your menu. Do you have a late night meeting or evening soccer practice for your child that week? Then include a Crock-Pot recipe for that night, or cook a large meal the night before and have leftovers the next day.

Chop and prepare a large variety and sufficient quantities of vegetables on your day off, and keep them in the refrigerator for easy access and use during the week. Many grocery stores now offer prewashed and precut vegetables, which can be used for your convenience as well. (Do rewash these yourself if planning to eat them raw).

Bulk cook your proteins and grains and store them in the refrigerator or freezer for later use during the week to make easy, delicious, quick meals.

Make double or triple portions of any meal to take for lunch the next day or to freeze for use as a ready meal on a night when you are not able to cook.

Prepare a variety of steamed and oven roasted vegetables in batches. They can be easily used to prepare salads and soups or can be added as a side dish to your main meals throughout the week.

Prepare your breakfast the night before if you don't have time to cook in the morning. You may choose an easy recipe for a slow cooker (i.e. oatmeal—recipe below) or soak chia seeds or oats in skim milk overnight and top it in the morning with your favorite berries and nuts for a delicious breakfast.

Batch-cook some legumes. Legumes are versatile and can be used in salads and side dishes or can be combined with vegetables to make delicious soups.

Prepare a few hard-boiled eggs, and keep them in your refrigerator. Eggs can be used for breakfast or added to salads and other dishes.

RECIPES

Some of the following recipes were shared by Kelly Ahearn[1], Andrea Beaman[2], Ellen Gavrielov[3] and Marcin Machula[4]

BREAKFAST

Cottage Cheese with Pineapple (1 serving) [4]

½ cup low-fat cottage cheese
1/4 cup freshly diced pineapple
1/4 cup diced mango
1 tablespoon chopped walnuts
1 tablespoon shredded coconut
1 tablespoon unsweetened cocoa powder (optional)

- Place the cottage cheese in a serving bowl.
- Mix in the pineapple, mango, and walnuts.
- Top with shredded coconut, sprinkle the cocoa powder, and serve immediately.

Option: Add a third of carrot, shredded.

<u>Slow Cooker Oats</u> (4 servings)

1 cup rolled oats
1 apple diced
A pinch of salt
1 cup of milk
1 cup of water
2 tablespoons of chopped walnuts and sunflower seeds
1 tablespoon of raisins
4 dry dates chopped
2 tablespoon of raw honey
2 tablespoons of butter

- Butter the slow cooker pan,
- Add a layer of apples, oats, and other ingredients, pour over milk and water.
- Cook on low heat for 6-8 hours. Garnish with berries before serving.

Overnight Oats (2 servings) [1]

1/2 cup rolled Oats
1 teaspoon of the following ingredients: raw cacao powder, acai powder, maca powder, spirulina powder and chia seeds
1 Tablespoon of goji berries or mulberries
1/4-1/2 cup Kefir (either regular or goats milk, plain)
2 tbsp of water
1 tbsp of wheat germ
1 tbsp of ground flax seed
1 square dark chocolate, 75% or higher
½ teaspoon of maple syrup
1 scoop nut butter of choice (natural no partially hydrogenated oils)
1 scoop plain strained yogurt such as Greek style
1 small banana

- Mix oats, powders, chia seeds, and berries with kefir and some water; mix well
- Top with wheat germ and flax seed
- Place dark chocolate square, nut butter, and yogurt on top of mixture
- Drizzle with maple syrup and place in fridge overnight
- In the morning slice one small banana on top and enjoy!

<u>Baked Eggocado</u> (1-2 servings)

1 medium ripe avocado
2 eggs
1 teaspoon of lemon juice
Salt and pepper as desired

- Cut avocado in half lengthwise and remove the pit.
- With the spoon scoop out a little bit of the avocado to make a bigger opening.
- Pour 1 egg in each avocado half, sprinkle with salt and pepper and bake in the oven at 200 degrees until the eggs are cooked.
- Drizzle with lemon juice if desired and serve immediately

<u>Zucchini Pancakes</u> (4 servings)[3]

2 medium zucchinis, coarsely shredded
1 teaspoon lemon zest
1 large garlic clove minced
½ teaspoon cumin
¼ teaspoon black pepper
½ cup whole wheat flower
½ teaspoon baking power
2 eggs, lightly beaten
2 tablespoons of olive oil

- Combine zucchini, lemon zest, garlic, cumin, salt, and peeper.
- Stir in the beaten eggs
- Add the baking powder and flower, mix thoroughly.
- Heat a lightly oiled griddle; scoop 2 tablespoons of batter onto the griddle.
- Cook on both sides and serve hot.

<u>Spinach Omelet</u> (2 servings)

4 eggs lightly beaten
¼ teaspoon salt and pepper
½ cup ricotta
½ cup of chopped spinach
2 medium tomatoes chopped
½ cup of mozzarella shredded

- Preheat oven to 300 degrees.
- Combine all the ingredients in a bowl;
- Grease a baking dish and spread the mixture evenly.
- Bake for 30 minutes until evenly baked, serve hot.

Parsley Smoothie (1 serving) [4]

1 ripe mango peeled and pitted
2 bananas
3 cups spinach
1 cup fresh Italian parsley
1 scoop almond butter
8 ounces water, coconut water or goats milk

- Put all ingredients in a blender with the fruit cut up and blend well.

Almond Butter and Apple Smoothie (2 Servings) [4]

2 apples, peeled and chopped
1/2 cup unsweetened apple cider or unfiltered apple juice
1/2 cup low-fat milk (rice, soy, or almond)
1 frozen banana
2 tablespoons peanut butter (or other nut butter)
2 tablespoons flaxseeds or flax oil
¼ teaspoon cinnamon
1/8 teaspoon cardamom
4 to 6 ice cubes

- Place all the ingredients in a blender and blend until smooth. Serve immediately.

<u>Blueberries and Cottage Cheese Smoothie</u> (4 servings) [4]

2 cups blueberries

2 mangoes

1/2 cup pomegranate juice

8 ounces low-fat cottage cheese

1 tablespoon maple syrup or honey

2 tablespoons golden flaxseeds

1/2 cup of ice cubes

- In a blender, mix the blueberries, pomegranate juice, mango, cottage cheese, maple syrup, flaxseeds, and ice. Serve immediately.

SALADS AND SIDE DISHES

<u>Spicy Edamame Hummus</u> (4 servings) [4]

Makes about 1 ½ cup

1 ½ cup frozen edamame
¼ cup tahini
2 tablespoons flaxseeds
2 tablespoons lime juice
2 garlic cloves, minced
1 teaspoon wasabi mustard (or less if milder flavor is desired)
Pinch of salt
Pinch of pepper
1 Tablespoon freshly minced cilantro
Water or vegetable stock
2 tablespoons olive oil

- Cook the edamame according to package instructions.
- In a food processor, puree the edamame, tahini, flaxseeds, lime juice, wasabi, salt, pepper, and cilantro.
- Add enough water or vegetable stock until desired thickness.
- Drizzle olive oil and mix before serving. It is best served cold.

Comments: Serve with vegetables such as carrots, celery, cucumber, or broccoli.

Shredded Zucchini Salad (4 servings) [4]

1 large green zucchini
1 large yellow squash
1 large carrot, peeled
1/2 shallot, minced
1 large garlic clove, minced
2 tablespoon lemon juice
1/2 teaspoon Dijon mustard
3 tablespoons olive oil
1 tablespoon freshly minced basil
1 tablespoon freshly minced Italian parsley
4 teaspoons freshly grated Parmesan cheese
Salt and pepper to taste

- Mix the shallot, garlic, lemon juice, mustard, olive oil, and herbs in a large bowl.
- Season with salt and pepper.
- Using a mandolin or shredder; shred the zucchini, squash, and carrot. Transfer to the bowl and mix.
- Divide among four plates, top with a little freshly grated Parmesan cheese, and serve immediately.

<u>Quick Healthy Cauliflower Casserole</u> (4 servings) [4]

1 tablespoon grape seed oil
1 slice whole wheat bread, toasted and grinded to small crumbs
2 tablespoons mixed salad herbs
1 cauliflower
Salt and pepper to taste

- Separate cauliflower florets and set aside.
- Bring to boil a steamer. Add the florets and cook until tender, about 10 minutes.
- Meanwhile mix the herbs with bread crumbs.
- Remove florets and transfer to a gratin dish.
- Mix in the oil, season to taste, and top with the bread crumbs mixture.
- Brown under a broiler until golden brown and serve immediately.

<u>Mushrooms and Raspberries Salad</u> (2 servings) [4]

1/2 cup baby spinach, cleaned

4 ounces mushrooms

1 tablespoon lemon juice

1 teaspoon grape seed oil

1/4 small sweet red onion, chopped

1 tablespoon raspberry vinegar

2 tablespoons walnut oil

2 teaspoons freshly minced salad herbs

2 tablespoons raspberries

2 teaspoons chopped walnuts

Salt and pepper to taste

- Peel the mushrooms and mix in with lemon juice.
- In a bowl mix the vinegar, walnut oil, and herbs. Season to taste and set aside.
- Heat the oil in a nonstick pan over medium heat. Add the mushrooms and sauté for 1 minute.
- Add the onion and continue to sauté for another minute.
- Remove from heat and mix in the vinaigrette.
- Equally divide the spinach and top with the mushrooms.
- Add the raspberries, walnuts, and serve immediately.

SNACKS

<u>Goat Cheese Log</u> (12 servings) [4]

1 – approx. 11 ounces plain goat cheese log
8 tablespoons medium coarse ground flaxseed
2 tablespoon paprika
1 tablespoon Cajun spices
4 tablespoons raw honey, warm

- Mix the flaxseed, paprika, and Cajun spices in a plate.
- Brush the warmed honey over the goat cheese log.
- Roll the log into the prepared mix. Refrigerate before use.

Could be served as an appetizer with small toasted slices of bread or vegetables slices, or to top a baby spinach salad with a slice of the goat cheese log

<u>Healthy Snack Mix</u>[4]

Coconut chips, unsweetened
Dry Roasted Mixed Nuts
Black Mulberries

- Take a generous amount of each and mix together.
- Place in individual bags or containers to bring with you on your travels

Crispy Cauliflower (4 servings)

1 head cauliflower
½ teaspoon salt and black pepper
1 oz of olive oil

- Preheat oven to 400 degrees.
- Cut cauliflower into small sized florets, sprinkle with salt, paper and drizzle with oil.
- Spread as one layer on a baking sheet and bake/roast in the oven for 25 minutes.

Kale Chips (4 servings)

1 packet of fresh kale
2 tablespoons of olive oil
½ teaspoon of salt

- Preheat oven to 350 degrees.
- Chop kale into bite size pieces removing the stem.
- Drizzle with olive oil and mix well to coat all the pieces.
- Spread as one layer on a baking sheet and bake/roast in the oven for 7-10 minutes on each side.
- Let them cool and sprinkle with salt.

Sweet Potato Chips (4 servings)

2 medium sweet potatoes well scrubbed and washed
2 tablespoon of olive oil
½ teaspoon ground cinnamon

- Preheat oven to 250° F.
- Cut sweet potatoes into thin slices and drizzle with olive oil.
- Spread as one layer on a baking sheet and bake/roast in the oven for 45-50 minutes on each side.
- Let them cool and sprinkle with cinnamon.

SOUPS AND MAIN DISHES

<u>Eggplant Potée</u> (4 servings) [4]

2 teaspoons olive oil

1 medium onion, diced

4 large garlic cloves, diced

1 medium eggplant, diced

1 large red bell pepper, diced

1 large tomato, peeled and diced

1 jalapeno, seeded and diced

2 tablespoons coconut milk

½ to 1 teaspoon cayenne pepper

1 tablespoon freshly minced Thai Basil

Salt to taste

- Heat the oil in a large saucepan over medium heat.
- Add the onion and sauté until translucent.
- Add the garlic and continue to cook for another minute.
- Add the eggplant, bell pepper, tomato, and jalapeno.
- Reduce heat, cover, and continue to cook for 15 minutes, stirring on occasion.
- Mix in the coconut milk and cayenne pepper.
- Continue to cook until liquid starts reduce or thicken.
- Add basil, salt to taste and serve immediately.

<u>Tilapia with Kumquat Sauce</u> (4 servings) [4]

2 teaspoons olive oil

4 – 4 ounces tilapia filets

2 teaspoons kumquat zest, minced

1 teaspoon orange zest, minced

1 teaspoon freshly minced ginger

1/2 cup freshly squeezed orange juice

7 kumquats cut in half

6 fresh Sweet Asian Basil leaves, minced

Cornstarch with water

Salt and pepper to taste

- Place the zests, ginger, orange juice, and half of the basil in a pan. Bring to boil over high heat.
- Add the kumquat halves and reduce the liquid by half.
- Thicken with a little bit of cornstarch water mixture, if desired.
- Heat a sauté pan with the olive oil over medium high heat.
- Add the fish and cook until golden brown.
- Turn-over and continue to cook until the fish flesh start to flake.
- Transfer to a serving platter, pour over the prepared sauce, sprinkle remaining basil, and serve immediately.

<u>Quinoa with Roasted Vegetables and Herbs</u> (6 to 8 servings) [4]

1 large eggplant, diced
1 large zucchini, diced
1 yellow bell pepper, diced
1 red bell pepper, diced
1 large red onion, diced
16 cherry tomatoes
8 cloves garlic, halved
2 sprigs fresh rosemary
2 bunches freshly minced basil
2 tablespoons olive oil
4 cups warm cooked quinoa
1 lemon
Salt and pepper

- Place the eggplant, zucchini, bell peppers, onion, and garlic in a bowl.
- Add 2 tablespoons olive oil, rosemary, ¾ of the minced basil and season to taste. Mix well and refrigerate for an hour.
- Preheat the barbecue on medium high. Transfer the vegetables to a barbecue vegetable pan.
- Roast over the fire until the vegetables are crunchy and slightly browned, mixing on occasion.
- Add the tomatoes and cook for another 2 minutes.
- Spread the warm quinoa in the bottom of a serving platter and top with the grilled vegetables. Sprinkle lemon juice, remaining basil and serve immediately.

<u>European Influenced Dinner</u> (1 serving) [1]

2 slices of German Rye Bread
1 tbsp Mustard
1 slice of cheddar, goat or sheep's cheese
3-4 ounces tuna in 1 tsp of olive
Salt and pepper
Handful of spinach or 2 leaves of leafy green vegetable
Cucumbers slices
1/2 avocado
1 tbsp hummus
Handful broccoli sprouts
Sliced red pepper

- Smear mustard on bread; add cheese, tuna, cucumber, sprouts and lettuce on top.
- Mash avocado with hummus, enjoy with sliced peppers
- This open-faced sandwich is a common dinner in Germany with the influence of other cultures using the avocado and hummus as a side dip. It is quick, healthy, simple and flavorful. This can be enjoyed cold or warmed in toaster oven.

<u>Chilled Cucumber and Salmon Soup</u> (2 servings) [4]

4 ounces cold sushi grade raw salmon, diced
1 large cucumber, peeled
1 small carrot, peeled
1/2 shallot
1 small garlic clove
1 teaspoon lemon juice
4 tablespoons low-fat Greek yogurt
2 tablespoons freshly minced dill
Salt and pepper to taste

- In a blender, liquefy the cucumber, carrot, shallot, garlic, lemon juice, and 1 tablespoon of dill.
- Season to taste and refrigerate. When cold, mix in the yogurt and then divide among two serving soup plates.
- Top each plate with 2 ounces diced salmon and sprinkle over a little of finely chopped dill. Serve immediately.

<u>Lentil Stew (Slow cooker preparation)</u> (4 servings) [2]

2 tablespoons of olive oil

1 Medium leek cut into 1-inch pieces

2 garlic cloves, peeled and minced

4 cups of stock or water

3 cups cooked lentils

2 parsnips, in ½-inch dice

3 carrots, in ½ inch dice

¼ teaspoon black pepper

1 medium celeriac root chopped in ½ inch dice

1 Yukon gold potato, in ½ inch dice

1 ½ teaspoons of salt

¼ cup minced parsley

- Put all ingredients except parsley into a slow cooker, and add 4 cups of water or stock.

- Cook on high heat for 4 hours or low heat for 8 hours.

- Garnish with parsley before serving.

<u>Stewed Lamb With Apricots</u> (4 servings) [2]

8-10 ounces of pastured lamb stew meat, cubed

2 tablespoons of olive oil

½ teaspoon cumin

½ teaspoon cinnamon

6-8 dried apricots, diced

¼ cup raisins

2 onions, peeled and quartered

3 garlic cloves chopped

½ teaspoon sea salt

1/8 teaspoon black pepper

1 cup water or stock

1 ½ cups red wine

1 sprig fresh parsley chopped

- Place ingredients into a slow cooker starting with olive oil at the bottom, onions, garlic, apricots, raisins, cumin, cinnamon, salt, pepper, 1 cup of stock, wine and the stew meat on top.
- Cook in slow cooker 4-5 hours on high temperature, or 8-10 hours on low.
- Garnish with parsley before serving

DESSERTS

<u>Baked Apples</u> (2 servings)

4 medium size apples

1 tablespoon of butter

2 tablespoons sunflower seeds

Two tablespoons chopped walnuts

1-tablespoon raw honey

- Preheat oven 300° F.

- Mix in a bowl butter, honey, walnuts and sunflower seeds.

- Fill scooped out apples with the filling and bake in the oven until tender for 20-30 minutes. Serve hot.

<u>Oatmeal Walnut Chocolate Chip Cookies</u> (4 servings) [2]

1 ½ cups rolled oats

½ cup whole grain flour

¼ teaspoon sea salt

1/3 cup granulated cane juice

½ cup walnuts, chopped

¼ cup dark chocolate chips

1 egg, beaten

3 tablespoons butter

1 tablespoons coconut oil

1 teaspoon vanilla extract

- Preheat oven to 350° F.
- Mix dry ingredients and wet ingredients in a separate bowl.
- Mix two of them into a batter.
- Line a baking pan with wax paper
- Scoop ½ tablespoon of butter onto baking sheet.
- Bake 18-20 minutes until golden brown

CONTRIBUTORS

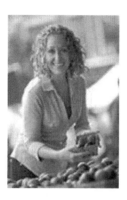

Andrea Beaman

Andrea Beaman is a Natural Foods Chef, thyroid expert and holistic health coach dedicated to alternative healing, and sustainable eating and living. Andrea was a featured contestant on Bravo's Top Chef. She is a regularly featured food and health expert on CBS News, and hosted the Award Nominated, Fed UP! A cooking show that educates viewers how to cook for, and cure, their bodily ailments. Andrea is recognized as one of the top 100 Most Influential People in Health and Fitness, and received the Award For Excellence in Health Supportive Food Education, as well the Health Leadership Award. She teaches engaging cooking demos and health programs to students and clients via live conferences, schools, and online programs, reaching people around the world. Andrea is the author of The Whole Truth – How I Naturally Reclaimed My Health, and You Can Too! and The Eating and Recipe Guide – Better Food, Better Health, and Health is Wealth – Make a Delicious Investment in You. Through her books, DVD's and live classes, Andrea makes learning about better health, good food, and a sustainable lifestyle a fun experience for everyone.

Website: www.AndreaBeaman.com

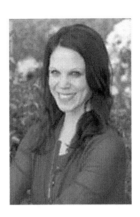

Kelly J. Ahearn, MS RDN, CDN

Kelly is a Registered Dietitian with a Master of Science degree in Nutrition and Dietetics from New York University. She holds a Bachelor of Science degree in Exercise Physiology from the University of Southern Maine and is a certified Pilates Teacher. She is a member of the Academy of Nutrition and Dietetics and is involved in Dietitians in Functional and Integrative Medicine, Nutrition Entrepreneurs, and Women's Health Dietetic Practice Groups, the Asian Indians in Nutrition and Dietetics Member Practice Group as well as a member of the American Society of Reproductive Medicine where she is actively involved in staying up-to-date on the latest research on fertility and achieving a healthy pregnancy through lifestyle factors. She has special interests in maternal nutrition and epigenetics, fertility and nutrition, PCOS, sports nutrition and integrative functional medicine. She is an avid believer in Joseph Pilates' "The Method" as the ultimate form of mind-body exercise and is a certified PAI teacger. Kelly is the Co-Founder of *Dietitians for Professional Integrity*, a not-for-profit organization of dietitians nationwide that believe the American public deserves nutrition information that is not tainted by food industry interests. She meets people where they are at and emphasizes the connection between food and cultural backgrounds.

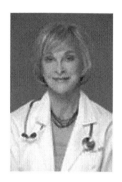

Hyla Cass, MD

Dr. Cass is Board-certified in psychiatry and neurology (ABPN) as well as integrative and holistic medicine (ABIHM), Dr. Cass is nationally recognized expert and educator in integrative medicine. She has appeared on The Dr. Oz Show, The View, numerous radio shows, and is widely quoted in national magazines. Author of several popular books including: Natural Highs, The Addicted Brain and How to Break Free, and 8 Weeks to Vibrant Health, she has also developed specialized nutritional supplements for addiction recovery as well as for enhancing mind, mood and energy. She has a clinical practice in Southern California. A well-known international speaker she also lectures to her medical colleagues on these same topics.

Web site: www.cassmd.com

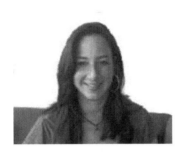

Dana Cohen, MD

Dr. Dana Cohen is renowned by her peers and beloved by patients for her nuanced practice of Integrative Medicine. In practice for over 15 years, she trained under the late Dr. Robert Atkins, author of the iconic Dr. Atkins' New Diet Revolution, and Dr. Ronald L. Hoffman, a pioneer of integrative medicine and founder of the Hoffman Center in New York City. She earned her MD from St. George's University School of Medicine and completed a three-year internal medicine residency at Albany Medical Center.

Dr. Cohen was certified by the American Board of Internal Medicine in 1998 and was recently appointed to the Board of Directors of the American College for the Advancement of Medicine (ACAM), the leading voice of Integrative Medicine for more than 1,500 MD, DO, ND and master-level health care providers, where she is also program director of their biyearly symposiums.

Website: http://www.drdanacohen.com

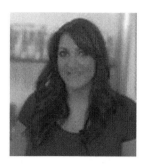

Ellen Gavrielov

Ellen Gavrielov is a cosmetology and aesthetic business consultant who specializes in marketing strategy development, guest experience and sales training in New York City. Ellen holds a Bachelor degree in Cosmetic and Fragrance marketing from the Fashion Institute of Technology. Upon her graduation in 2008, Ellen has been using her expertise in product formulations to help educate consumers on how to properly purchase the right products for their skincare needs based on the ingredients used. She strongly believes that cosmetic products must be formulated with high quality plant extracts in order to reap the full benefits of the product. Ellen focuses on the holistic approach towards treating skin. Her fundamental goal is to educate consumers on the many benefits of consuming an organic diet both inside and out to help preserve the skin and radiate beauty.

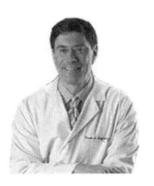

Ronald Hoffman, MD

Dr. Ronald Hoffman is an American physician, author, and broadcaster who hosts Intelligent Medicine, a syndicated radio talk show, and the Intelligent Medicine Podcast. He is the founder and director of the Hoffman Center in New York City, and is a practitioner of holistic medicine. Dr. Hoffman is recognized as one of America's foremost complementary medicine practitioners. He is author of numerous books and articles for the public and for health professionals. He is active in several medical professional organizations, and is a past President of the country's largest organization of complementary and alternative doctors, the American College for Advancement in Medicine (ACAM). He is a frequent guest on radio and TV, and is frequently quoted in popular magazines and newspapers. He is also called upon to lecture both to the public and to groups of medical professionals. On the personal side, his active lifestyle is an embodiment of the healthy principles he espouses.

Website: http://drhoffman.com/

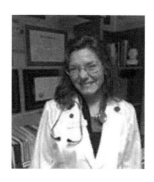

Nancy Iankowitz, DNP

Dr. Nancy Iankowitz is a Doctor of Nursing Practice (DNP), and ANCC Board certified as an Advanced Practice Registered Nurse (APRN) since 1984. For over 29 years, she has enjoyed incorporating into her practice a multidisciplinary approach (including Reiki, therapeutic touch, guided imagery and other healing modalities from both eastern as well as western inspired disciplines). As a certified Reiki Healer for over ten years, she has great respect for an integrative approach to wellness. Dr. Iankowitz is former research coordinator of the AECOM Longevity Genes Project, former Associate Director of Nursing, and former Director of Care Management at a large community health organization. She enjoys teaching nursing students at both the college and university levels, is licensed in New York State and Connecticut, adjunct faculty in the Division of Nursing at Mount Saint Mary College in Newburgh, NY, an active member of the Mu Epsilon Chapter of Sigma Theta Tau International Honor Society, and is the Director of Holistic and Integrative Healing LLC.

Website: www.neciankowitz.com

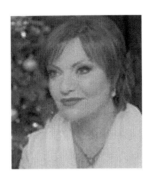

Svetlana Kotlovskiy

Svetlana Kotlovskiy is a Certified Laser Specialist, Licensed Cosmetologist and a Director of Green Planet Spa in New York. Svetlana holds a Bachelor degree in Commerce and Economics from Ukranian National University and a Diploma in Aesthetics and Cosmetology from Elite Academy of Beauty Arts. Svetlana became a Director of Green Planet Spa in 2009, one of the first places that offer a painless laser hair removal treatment by ALMA Laser Soprano technology. Under Svetlana's expert supervision Green Planet Spa expanded and now provides different services including a variety of hair and nail treatments, laser hair removal services and esthetics procedures. Svetlana is passionate about helping women to look and feel their best using nurturing and most natural products. Green Planet Spa offers hair strengthening treatment with Nanomax and hair nurturing color technology with INOA. Esthetic services are provided utilizing products from Osmosis Pur skincare line, which is based on natural antioxidants and botanical extracts.

Website: http://www.gphairsalonanddayspabrooklyn.com/

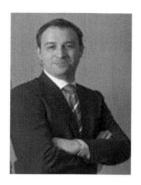

Arkady Aaron Lipnitsky, DC, DACRB, CICE

Dr. Arkady Lipnitsky is a Diplomat of the American Chiropractic Rehabilitation Board and Director of Chiropractic and Rehabilitation at Pain Physicians New York. He also holds postgraduate Certifications from Dry Needling Institute and Certification in Manipulation Under Anesthesia. He is a Fellow of International Society for Medical Shockwave Treatment and one of leading specialists in Shockwave therapy of sport injuries and soft tissue traumas.

Dr. Lipnitsky actively participates in research and development of a new age multi-spectral laser technology and its diverse application in treatment of many neuromusculoskeletal conditions. He is a creator of a popular instructional exercise video "Lower Back and Pelvis Mobility and Core Stability Training". Dr. Lipnitsky utilizes many techniques and treatment protocols like ART, FMS, Eccentric exercise training, Spinal Decompression, gentle spinal manipulation techniques, Kinesis One and Vibra-Core training. Throughout the years, Dr. Lipnitsky has developed truly unique treatment protocols, combining his advanced Eastern European massage skills with his diverse experience in Chiropractic medicine and Functional Rehabilitation to treat some of the most challenging neuromuscular and skeletal conditions.

Website: www.painfreenyc.com

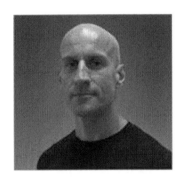

Marcin Machula, PES

Marcin Machula is Performance Enhancement Specialist and Corrective Exercise Specialist. He is founder of "The MMX Performance"; he is dedicated to excellence and innovations in sports performance and strength development. Marcin Machula began his interest in physical training, boxing, kickboxing, and weight training at the early age of sixteen. In 1992, he joined "The French Foreign Legion" and he was among the elite endurance performers in the 2nd Infantry regiment, Nimes, France. While in The Foreign Legion he was awarded with the prestigious TOP RUN (Cross County) award. He took part in annual marathons and half marathons in Castelnaudary, France. Marcin brings 20-plus years of experience to his clients in order to help them reach their fitness goals. He has worked with many levels of clients,   from post-injury to actors and models to athletes who compete at all levels of sporting events. Recognizing that each person is unique, he doesn't believe in "cookie cutter "programs. He personally customizes individual programs, and provides the hands on coaching and motivation necessary to make a lasting and visible change in client's life.

Website: http://www.mmxperformance.com/

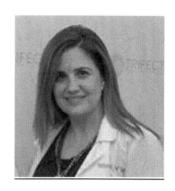

Inna Natkovitch

Inna Natkovitch is a Licensed Medical Esthetician, a Licensed Cosmetologist and a Certified Laser Specialist. Inna holds a Diploma in Aesthetics and Cosmetology from College of Cosmetology and Esthetics from Russian National Fabomed Institute. Inna is a caring and compassioned esthetician with more than 20 years of experience in performing a wide range of facial and skincare services. Her vast knowledge and experience includes performing a wide variety of professional services such as Microdermabrasions, HydraFacials, Laser Hair Removal, Vela Shape, CoolSculpting and Zerona Cellulite and Fat Reduction, Laser Skin Rejuvenation and Tightening, Silk Peel Dermalinfusion, Meta Therapy and Ultherapy among others. Inna believes that it is important to educate people on the benefits of being healthy both inside and out. Inna utilizes both science and nature to provide result-oriented and personalized treatments for acne –prone, photo-damaged, aging and sensitive skin to restore skin's health by using the freshest technology and ingredients customized to each client's needs.

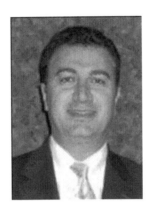

Dr. Daniel Roshan, MD

Dr. Daniel Roshan is a Board-certified OB/GYN, Maternal-Fetal Medicine (high-risk OB/GYN) specialist. He is an active member of the American College of Ob/Gyn and American College of Surgeons. He was trained at Johns Hopkins hospital and is a member of Johns Hopkins Medical and Surgical Society, Johns Hopkins Howard Kelly Society, Society for Maternal-Fetal Medicine, American Society for Human Genetics, Society for Gynecologic investigation, Bellevue Ob/Gyn Society and New York Obstetrics Society.

He is a founder of the Sephardic American Medical Society. He has published over 50 research abstracts and presented original research papers at many scientific societies such as: Society for Gynecological Investigation, Society for Maternal-Fetal Medicine, American college of Ob/Gyn and American Institute for Ultrasound in Medicine. He has performed or supervised over 10,000 births, 6,000 amniocenteses, and over 2,000 Chorionic Villus samplings. He gets referrals from all over the country for Chorionic villus sampling (CVS) and actively lectures and teaches this procedure. He is also expert in recurrent pregnancy losses, Thrombophilia and pregnancy such as factor V Laiden mutation, Prot S and C deficiency, Diabetes in pregnancy, Thyroid disease in pregnancy, seizure disorders, pre-term labor and multiple pregnancies such as twins, triplets, and quadruplets. He has performed many cerclage procedures. He considers it an honor and a priviledge to take care of a high-risk patient.

Website: http://www.roshmfm.com/

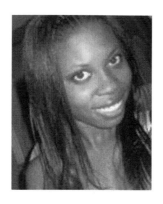

Andrea Small

Born in Los Angeles, California and raised in Florida, Andrea started drawing from the moment she could pick up a pencil. She's always had a passion for creativity and drawing. In 1997 at the age of 8, Andrea entered an art contest and placed second. Throughout grade school, Andrea has entered many drawing contest and has had her work on display. In 2001 at the age of 14, Andrea won 'Best Display' at the World's Fair at Carver Middle School in Delray Beach, Florida. She created a life size tepee with the help of her twin sister. Andrea pursued an art career at Miami International University of Art & Design and graduated with a Bachelor's of Fine Arts in Computer Animation in 2011 but specializes in Illustrations and concept drawings. Andrea relocated to New York City in late 2013 where she currently resides and Free-lances.

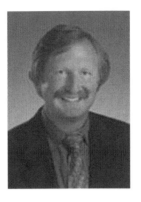

Jacob Teitelbaum, MD

Dr. Jacob Teitelbaum is Director of the Practitioners Alliance Network and author of the popular free iPhone &Android application "Cures A-Z," and of the best-selling book From Fatigued to Fantastic!, Pain Free 1-2-3—A Proven Program for Eliminating Chronic Pain Now, the Beat Sugar Addiction NOW! Series, Real Cause, Real Cure, and The Fatigue and Fibromyalgia Solution. He is the lead author of 4 studies on effective treatment for fibromyalgia and chronic fatigue syndrome, and a study on effective treatment of autism using NAET. Dr. Teitelbaum does frequent media appearances including Good Morning America, CNN, Fox News Channel, the Dr Oz Show and Oprah & Friends. He lives in Kona, Hawaii.

Web site: www.EndFatigue.com

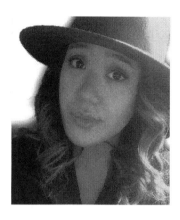

Julia Lin

Born in New York City, Julia is currently pursuing a career in Interior Architecture at Pratt Institute. Julia studied the understanding between spatial conditions and typographic characteristics. She is currently working on personal projects involving Responsive Web Design while simultaneously attending school for her Bachelor's in Interior Architecture. She currently resides in New York City and is available for freelance.

REFERENCES

CALMING YOUR MIND

1.   Dahlstrom, Alexandrea. "Modern Meditation." At the Lake (2015): 94. Web. 12 Apr. 2015.

2.   Goyal, Madhav, Sonal Singh, Erica M S Sibinga, Neda F. Gould, Anastasia Rowland-Seymour, Ritu Sharma, Zackary Berger, Dana Sleicher, David D. Maron, Hasan M. Shihab, Padmini D. Ranasinghe, Shauna Linn, Shonali Saha, Eric B. Bass, and Jennifer A. Haythornthwaite. "Meditation Programs for Psychological Stress and Well-being: A Systematic Review and Meta-analysis." JAMA Internal Medicine 174.3 (2014): 357-68. Web. 12 Apr. 2015.

3.   Gyatso, Kelsang. Transform Your Life: A   Blissful Journey. London: Tharpa Publications, 2001. Print.

4.   "What Meditation Can Do for Your Mind, Mood, and Health. Taking a Few Minutes to Focus Your Mind Each Day Can Reduce Stress, Pain, Depression, and More." Harvard Women's Health Watch 21.12 (2014): 6. Web. 12 Apr. 2015.

5.   "The Chopra Center." Chopra.com. N.p., n.d. Web. 12 Apr. 2015

6.   Dahlstrom, Alexandrea. "Modern Meditation." *At the Lake* (2015): 94. *MasterFILE Complete*. Web. 25 Nov. 2015.

7.   Goyal, Madhav, Sonal Singh, Erica M S Sibinga, Neda F. Gould, Anastasia Rowland-Seymour, Ritu Sharma, Zackary Berger, Dana Sleicher, David D. Maron, Hasan M. Shihab, Padmini D. Ranasinghe, Shauna Linn, Shonali Saha, Eric B. Bass, and Jennifer A. Haythornthwaite. "Meditation Programs for Psychological Stress and Well-being: A Systematic Review and Meta-analysis." *JAMA Internal Medicine* 174.3 (2014): 357-68. *MEDLINE Complete*. Web. 25 Nov. 2015.

8. "Book of All Quotes." Book of All Quotes. N.p., n.d. Web. 13oct.2015, http://www.bookofallquotes.com/

REDEFINING YOUR MIND — THE ART OF SELF-AWARENESS

1. Allan, Blake A., Ryan D. Duffy, and Richard Douglass. "Meaning in Life and Work: A Developmental Perspective." *Journal of Positive Psychology* 10.4 (2015): 323-31 9p. *Ccm.* Web. 25 Nov. 2015.

2. Morin, Alain. "Self-Awareness Part 1: Definition, Measures, Effects, Functions, and Antecedents." *Social & Personality Psychology Compass* 5.10 (2011): 807-23. *Academic Search Complete.* Web. 25 Nov. 2015.

3. Pawlik-Kienlen, Laurie. "Live with Purpose." *Alive* 384 (2014): 43. *MasterFILE Complete.* Web. 25 Nov. 2015.

4. Vago, David R. "Mapping Modalities of Self-awareness in Mindfulness Practice: A Potential Mechanism for Clarifying Habits of Mind." *Annals of the New York Academy of Sciences* 1307.1 (2014): 28-42. *Academic Search Complete.* Web. 25 Nov. 2015.

5. "Book of All Quotes." Book of All Quotes. N.p., n.d. Web. 13oct.2015, http://www.bookofallquotes.com/

PART II — HEALING THE BODY

BALANCING A WOMAN'S HORMONAL ORCHESTRA

1. Barker, Liz. "Adrenal BurnOUT." Delicious Living 24.1 (2008): 51-53. Web. 29 Mar. 2015.

2. Begley, Sharon. "Stress." Saturday Evening Post 283.6 (2011): 36-37. Web. 29 Mar. 2015.

3. Berga, Sarah, and Frederick Naftolin. "Neuroendocrine Control of Ovulation." Gynecological Endocrinology: The Official Journal

Of The International Society Of Gynecological Endocrinology 28 Suppl 1 (2012): 9-13. Web. 29 Mar. 2015.

4.   Bradshaw-Black, V. "The Nutrition Maze: Nutritional Aspects of Adrenal Fatigue." Positive Health 156 (2009): 1. Web. 29 Mar. 2015.

5.   C. Stephens, Mary Ann1, and Gary2 Wand. "Stress and the HPA Axis." Alcohol Research: Current Reviews 34.4 (2012): 468-83. Web. 29 Mar. 2015.

6.   Cass, Hyla, and Kathleen Barnes. 8 Weeks to Vibrant Health: A Take-charge Plan for Women to Correct Imbalances, Reclaim Energy, and Restore Well-being. Brevard, NC: Take Charge, 2008. Print.

7.   Case Study of Ms Kl - Adrenal Fatigue. 28 Australasian College of Nutritional & Environmental Medicine Journal 14-15. N.d. Web.

8.   Charlesworth, Jenny. "RUNNING on Empty." Today's Parent 31.7 (2014): 30. Web. 29 Mar. 2015.

9.   Chi, Tsu-Tsair. "Curcuma, Cyperus and Astragalus: Herbs for Estrogen Dominance. An Initial in Vivo Study." Nutritional Perspectives: Journal of the Council on Nutrition 36.2 (2013): 33-38. Web. 29 Mar. 2015.

10.   Dedovic, Katarina, Catherine D'Aguiar, and Jens C. Pruessner. "What Stress Does to Your Brain: A Review of Neuroimaging Studies." Canadian Journal of Psychiatry 54.1 (2009): 6-15. Web. 29 Mar. 2015.

11.   Duclos, M., B. Gatta, J.-B. Corcuff, M. Rashedi, F. Pehourcq, and P. Roger. "Fat Distribution in Obese Women Is Associated with Subtle Alterations of the Hypothalamic–pituitary–adrenal Axis Activity and Sensitivity to Glucocorticoids." Clinical Endocrinology 55.4 (2001): 447-54. Web. 29 Mar. 2015.

12.   Farage, Miranda A., Thomas W. Osborn, and Allan B. Maclean. "Cognitive, Sensory, and Emotional Changes Associated with the

Menstrual Cycle: A Review." Archives Of Gynecology And Obstetrics 278.4 (2008): 299-307. Web. 29 Mar. 2015.

13. Fitzgerald, Kara. "Health Regimen for a 29-your-old Female Diagnosed with Adrenal Fatigue." Integrative Medicine: A Clinician's Journal 10.6 (2011): 36-42. Web. 29 Mar. 2015.

14. Fucic, Aleksandra, Marija Gamulin, Zeljko Ferencic, Jelena Katic, Martin Krayer Von Krauss, Alena Bartonova, and Domenico F. Merlo. "Environmental Exposure to Xenoestrogens and Oestrogen Related Cancers: Reproductive System, Breast, Lung, Kidney, Pancreas, and Brain." Environmental Health: A Global Access Science Source 11.Suppl 1 (2012): 1-8. Web. 29 Mar. 2015.

15. Giles, Grace E., Caroline R. Mahoney, Tad T. Brunyé, Holly A. Taylor, and Robin B. Kanarek. "Stress Effects on Mood, HPA Axis, and Autonomic Response: Comparison of Three Psychosocial Stress Paradigms." PLoS ONE 9.12 (2014): 1-19. Web. 29 Mar. 2015.

16. Greer, Michael. "Herbal Options for Managing Adrenal Fatigue." Holistic Primary Care 12.4 (2011): 5-6. Web. 29 Mar. 2015.

17. Gutman, David A., Alisa R. Gutman, Michael J. Owens, and Charles B. Nemeroff. "Stress Neurobiology and Corticotropin-Releasing Factor." Psychiatric Times 23.10 (2006): 91-95. Web. 29 Mar. 2015.

18. Head, Kathleen A., and Gregory S. Kelly. "Nutrients and Botanicals for Treatment of Stress: Adrenal Fatigue, Neurotransmitter Imbalance, Anxiety, and Restless Sleep." Alternative Medicine Review 14.2 (2009): 114-40. Web. 29 Mar. 2015.

19. Holtorf, K. "Diagnosis and Treatment of Hypothalamic-pituitary-adrenal (HPA) Axis Dysfunction in Patients with Chronic Fatigue Syndrome (CFS) and Fibromyalgia (FM)." Journal of Chronic Fatigue Syndrome 14.3 (2007): 59-88. Web. 29 Mar. 2015.

20. Hoyer, Jana, Inga Burmann, Marie-Luise Kieseler, Florian Vollrath, Lydia Hellrung, Katrin Arelin, Elisabeth Roggenhofer, Arno Villringer, and Julia Sacher. "Menstrual Cycle Phase Modulates Emotional Conflict Processing in Women with and without Premenstrual Syndrome (PMS) – A Pilot Study." PLoS ONE 8.4 (2013): 1-8. Web. 29 Mar. 2015.

21. Jang, Su Hee, Dong Il Kim, and Min-Sun Choi. "Effects and Treatment Methods of Acupuncture and Herbal Medicine for Premenstrual Syndrome/premenstrual Dysphoric Disorder: Systematic Review." BMC Complementary And Alternative Medicine 14 (2014): 11. Web. 29 Mar. 2015.

22. Khalsa, Kps. "Avert Adrenal Fatigue." Better Nutrition 70.10 (2008): 28. Web. 29 Mar. 2015.

23. Kiesner, Jeff, and Vincent T. Martin. "Mid-Cycle Headaches and Their Relationship to Different Patterns of Premenstrual Stress Symptoms." Headache: The Journal of Head & Face Pain 53.6 (2013): 935-46. Web. 29 Mar. 2015.

24. Kim, S-Y, H-J Park, H. Lee, and H. Lee. "Acupuncture for Premenstrual Syndrome: A Systematic Review and Meta-analysis of Randomised Controlled Trials." BJOG: An International Journal Of Obstetrics And Gynaecology 118.8 (2011): 899-915. Web. 29 Mar. 2015.

25. Kloss, Beth, A., Lisa, A. Marcom, Ann, M. Odom, Courtney, L. Tuggle, and Deborah Weatherspoon. "PMS Treatment Through the Use of CAM." International Journal of Childbirth Education 27.3 (2012): 60-64. Web. 29 Mar. 2015.

26. Klump, Kelly L., Pamela K. Keel, Sarah E. Racine, S. Alexandra Burt, Michael Neale, Cheryl L. Sisk, Steven Boker, and Jean Yueqin Hu. "The Interactive Effects of Estrogen and Progesterone on Changes in Emotional Eating across the Menstrual Cycle." Journal of Abnormal Psychology 122.1 (2013): 131-37. Web. 29 Mar. 2015.

27. Kumari, Veena, Joanna Konstantinou, Andrew Papadopoulos, Ingrid Aasen, Lucia Poon, Rozmin Halari, and Anthony J. Cleare. "Evidence for a Role of Progesterone in Menstrual Cycle-related Variability in Prepulse Inhibition in Healthy Young Women." Neuropsychopharmacology 35.4 (2010): 929-37. Web. 29 Mar. 2015.

28. La Rosa, Piergiorgio, Marco Pellegrini, Pierangela Totta, Filippo Acconcia, and Maria Marino. "Xenoestrogens Alter Estrogen Receptor (ER) α Intracellular Levels." PLoS ONE 9.2 (2014): 1-8. Web. 29 Mar. 2015.

29. Maniam, Jayanthi, Christopher Antoniadis, and Margaret J. Morris. "Early-life Stress, HPA Axis Adaptation, and Mechanisms Contributing to Later Health Outcomes." Frontiers in Endocrinology 5 (2014): 1-17. Web. 29 Mar. 2015.

30. "Mind over Matter." Diva 211 (2014): 62-63. Web. 29 Mar. 2015.

31. Minkel, Jared, Marisa Moreta, Julianne Muto, Oo Htaik, Christopher Jones, Mathias Basner, and David Dinges. "Sleep Deprivation Potentiates HPA Axis Stress Reactivity in Healthy Adults." Health Psychology 33.11 (2014): 1430-434. Web. 29 Mar. 2015.

32. Mosteller, R. "Adrenal Fatigue." Better Nutrition 70.6 (2008): 14. Web. 29 Mar. 2015.

33. Murray, Michael, T. "Fend off Adrenal Fatigue." Better Nutrition 76.7 (2014): 24-26. Web. 29 Mar. 2015.

34. Ochedalski, T., S. Subburaju, P. C. Wynn, and G. Aguilera. "Interaction between Oestrogen and Oxytocin on Hypothalamic-pituitary-adrenal Axis Activity." Journal of Neuroendocrinology 19.3 (2007): 189-97. Web. 29 Mar. 2015.

35. Pranjić, Nurka, Sabina Nuhbegović, Sanja Brekalo-Lazarević, and Azra Kurtić. "Is Adrenal Exhaustion Synonym of Syndrome

Burnout at Workplace?" Collegium Antropologicum 36.3 (2012): 911-19. Web. 29 Mar. 2015.

36. Rapkin, Andrea J., and Alin L. Akopians. "Pathophysiology of Premenstrual Syndrome and Premenstrual Dysphoric Disorder." Menopause International 18.2 (2012): 52-59. Web. 29 Mar. 2015.

37. Spiteri, Thierry, Sergei Musatov, Sonoko Ogawa, Ana Ribeiro, Donald W. Pfaff, and Anders Ågmo. "Estrogen-induced Sexual Incentive Motivation, Proceptivity and Receptivity Depend on a Functional Estrogen Receptor α in the Ventromedial Nucleus of the Hypothalamus but Not in the Amygdala." Neuroendocrinology 91.2 (2010): 142-54. Web. 29 Mar. 2015.

38. Sundström-Poromaa, Inger. "Action of Progesterone and Progesterone Metabolites in Menstrual-Cycle–Related Disorders." Headache: The Journal of Head & Face Pain 48 (2008): S90-98. Web. 29 Mar. 2015.

39. Tanriverdi, F., Z. Karaca, K. Unluhizarci, and F. Kelestimur. "The Hypothalamo-pituitary-adrenal Axis in Chronic Fatigue Syndrome and Fibromyalgia Syndrome." Stress: The International Journal on the Biology of Stress 10.1 (2007): 13-25. Web. 29 Mar. 2015.

40. Teepker, M., M. Peters, H. Vedder, K. Schepelmann, and S. Lautenbacher. "Menstrual Variation in Experimental Pain: Correlation with Gonadal Hormones." Neuropsychobiology 61.3 (2010): 131-40. Web. 29 Mar. 2015.

41. Turner, Lisa. "Find Hormonal Harmony & Counteract Xenoestrogens Naturally." Better Nutrition 71.5 (2009): 34. Web. 29 Mar. 2015.

42. Zhang, Die, Shen Yang, Chunhao Yang, Guozhang Jin, and Xuechu Zhen. "Estrogen Regulates Responses of Dopamine

Neurons in the Ventral Tegmental Area to Cocaine." Psychopharmacology 199.4 (2008): 625-35. Web. 29 Mar. 2015.

43. Zhang, Wanglong, Yu Luo, Li Zhang, Qian Cai, and Xuejun Pan. "Known and Emerging Factors Modulating Estrogenic Effects of Endocrine-disrupting Chemicals." Environmental Reviews 22.1 (2014): 87-98. Web. 29 Mar. 2015.

44. "Book of All Quotes." Book of All Quotes. N.p., n.d. Web. 13oct.2015, http://www.bookofallquotes.com/

THYROID GLAND -YOUR ENERGY MACHINE

1. Canaris G, Tape T, Wigton R. Thyroid disease awareness is associated with high rates of identifying subjects with previously undiagnosed thyroid dysfunction. BMC Public Health [serial online]. 2013;13:351. Available from: CINAHL Complete, Ipswich, MA. Accessed March 24, 2015.

2. Choi W, Kim J. Dietary factors and the risk of thyroid cancer: a review. Clinical Nutrition Research [serial online]. July 2014;3(2):75-88. Available from: MEDLINE Complete, Ipswich, MA. Accessed March 24, 2015.

3. Cléro É, Doyon F, de Vathaire F, et al. Dietary patterns, goitrogenic food, and thyroid cancer: a case-control study in French Polynesia. Nutrition And Cancer [serial online]. 2012;64(7):929-936. Available from: MEDLINE Complete, Ipswich, MA. Accessed March 24, 2015.

4. D'Adamo C, Sahin A. Soy foods and supplementation: a review of commonly perceived health benefits and risks. Alternative Therapies In Health And Medicine [serial online]. 2014 Winter 2014;20 Suppl 1:39-51. Available from: MEDLINE Complete, Ipswich, MA. Accessed March 24, 2015.

5. Doerge D, Chang H. Inactivation of thyroid peroxidase by soy isoflavones, in vitro and in vivo. Journal Of Chromatography. B,

Analytical Technologies In The Biomedical And Life Sciences [serial online]. September 25, 2002;777(1-2):269-279. Available from: MEDLINE Complete, Ipswich, MA. Accessed March 24, 2015.

6. Eichelsdoerfer P. Prescribing compounded bioidentical hormones: antiaging applications. Integrative Medicine: A Clinician's Journal [serial online]. June 2008;7(3):42-48. Available from: CINAHL Complete, Ipswich, MA. Accessed March 24, 2015.

7. Gunder L, Haddow S. Laboratory evaluation of thyroid function. Clinical Advisor [serial online]. December 2009;12(12):26. Available from: CINAHL Complete, Ipswich, MA. Accessed March 24, 2015.

8. Helmreich D, Parfitt D, Lu X, Akil H, Watson S. Relation between the hypothalamic-pituitary-thyroid (HPT) axis and the hypothalamic-pituitary-adrenal (HPA) axis during repeated stress. Neuroendocrinology [serial online]. 2005;81(3):183-192. Available from: MEDLINE Complete, Ipswich, MA. Accessed March 24, 2015.

9. Messina M, Redmond G. Effects of soy protein and soybean isoflavones on thyroid function in healthy adults and hypothyroid patients: a review of the relevant literature. Thyroid: Official Journal Of The American Thyroid Association [serial online]. March 2006;16(3):249-258. Available from: MEDLINE Complete, Ipswich, MA. Accessed March 24, 2015.

10. Ochs N, Auer R, Rodondi N, et al. Meta-analysis: subclinical thyroid dysfunction and the risk for coronary heart disease and mortality. Annals Of Internal Medicine [serial online]. June 3, 2008;148(11):832-845. Available from: CINAHL Complete, Ipswich, MA. Accessed March 24, 2015.

11. Rosen J, Gardiner P, Lee S, et al. Complementary and alternative medicine use among patients with thyroid cancer. Thyroid: Official Journal Of The American Thyroid Association [serial online]. October 2013;23(10):1238-1246. Available from: MEDLINE Complete, Ipswich, MA. Accessed March 24, 2015.

12. Rugge J, Bougatsos C, Chou R. Screening and treatment of thyroid dysfunction: an evidence review for the u.s. Preventive services task force. Annals Of Internal Medicine [serial online]. 2015 Jan 6 6, 2015;162(1):35-45. Available from: CINAHL Complete, Ipswich, MA. Accessed March 24, 2015.

13. "Book of All Quotes." Book of All Quotes. N.p., n.d. Web. 13oct.2015, http://www.bookofallquotes.com/

OVARIES MESSENGERS FROM VENUS

1. Berga, Sarah, and Frederick Naftolin. "Neuroendocrine Control of Ovulation." Gynecological Endocrinology: The Official Journal Of The International Society Of Gynecological Endocrinology 28 Suppl 1 (2012): 9-13. Web. 29 Mar. 2015.

2. Chi, Tsu-Tsair. "Curcuma, Cyperus and Astragalus: Herbs for Estrogen Dominance. An Initial in Vivo Study." Nutritional Perspectives: Journal of the Council on Nutrition 36.2 (2013): 33-38. Web. 29 Mar. 2015.

3. Farage, Miranda A., Thomas W. Osborn, and Allan B. Maclean. "Cognitive, Sensory, and Emotional Changes Associated with the Menstrual Cycle: A Review." Archives Of Gynecology And Obstetrics 278.4 (2008): 299-307. Web. 29 Mar. 2015.

4. Fucic, Aleksandra, Marija Gamulin, Zeljko Ferencic, Jelena Katic, Martin Krayer Von Krauss, Alena Bartonova, and Domenico F. Merlo. "Environmental Exposure to Xenoestrogens and Oestrogen Related Cancers: Reproductive System, Breast, Lung, Kidney, Pancreas, and Brain." Environmental Health: A Global Access Science Source 11.Suppl 1 (2012): 1-8. Web. 29 Mar. 2015.

5. Hoyer, Jana, Inga Burmann, Marie-Luise Kieseler, Florian Vollrath, Lydia Hellrung, Katrin Arelin, Elisabeth Roggenhofer, Arno Villringer, and Julia Sacher. "Menstrual Cycle Phase Modulates Emotional Conflict Processing in Women with and without

Premenstrual Syndrome (PMS) – A Pilot Study." PLoS ONE 8.4 (2013): 1-8. Web. 29 Mar. 2015.

6. Jang, Su Hee, Dong Il Kim, and Min-Sun Choi. "Effects and Treatment Methods of Acupuncture and Herbal Medicine for Premenstrual Syndrome/premenstrual Dysphoric Disorder: Systematic Review." BMC Complementary And Alternative Medicine 14 (2014): 11. Web. 29 Mar. 2015.

7. Kiesner, Jeff, and Vincent T. Martin. "Mid-Cycle Headaches and Their Relationship to Different Patterns of Premenstrual Stress Symptoms." Headache: The Journal of Head & Face Pain 53.6 (2013): 935-46. Web. 29 Mar. 2015.

8. Kim, S-Y, H-J Park, H. Lee, and H. Lee. "Acupuncture for Premenstrual Syndrome: A Systematic Review and Meta-analysis of Randomised Controlled Trials." BJOG: An International Journal Of Obstetrics And Gynaecology 118.8 (2011): 899-915. Web. 29 Mar. 2015.

9. Kloss, Beth, A., Lisa, A. Marcom, Ann, M. Odom, Courtney, L. Tuggle, and Deborah Weatherspoon. "PMS Treatment Through the Use of CAM." International Journal of Childbirth Education 27.3 (2012): 60-64. Web. 29 Mar. 2015.

10. Klump, Kelly L., Pamela K. Keel, Sarah E. Racine, S. Alexandra Burt, Michael Neale, Cheryl L. Sisk, Steven Boker, and Jean Yueqin Hu. "The Interactive Effects of Estrogen and Progesterone on Changes in Emotional Eating across the Menstrual Cycle." Journal of Abnormal Psychology 122.1 (2013): 131-37. Web. 29 Mar. 2015.

11. Kumari, Veena, Joanna Konstantinou, Andrew Papadopoulos, Ingrid Aasen, Lucia Poon, Rozmin Halari, and Anthony J. Cleare. "Evidence for a Role of Progesterone in Menstrual Cycle-related Variability in Prepulse Inhibition in Healthy Young Women." Neuropsychopharmacology 35.4 (2010): 929-37. Web. 29 Mar. 2015.

12. La Rosa, Piergiorgio, Marco Pellegrini, Pierangela Totta, Filippo Acconcia, and Maria Marino. "Xenoestrogens Alter Estrogen

Receptor (ER) α Intracellular Levels." PLoS ONE 9.2 (2014): 1-8. Web. 29 Mar. 2015.

13. Ochedalski, T., S. Subburaju, P. C. Wynn, and G. Aguilera. "Interaction between Oestrogen and Oxytocin on Hypothalamic-pituitary-adrenal Axis Activity." Journal of Neuroendocrinology 19.3 (2007): 189-97. Web. 29 Mar. 2015.

14. Rapkin, Andrea J., and Alin L. Akopians. "Pathophysiology of Premenstrual Syndrome and Premenstrual Dysphoric Disorder." Menopause International 18.2 (2012): 52-59. Web. 29 Mar. 2015.

15. Spiteri, Thierry, Sergei Musatov, Sonoko Ogawa, Ana Ribeiro, Donald W. Pfaff, and Anders Ågmo. "Estrogen-induced Sexual Incentive Motivation, Proceptivity and Receptivity Depend on a Functional Estrogen Receptor α in the Ventromedial Nucleus of the Hypothalamus but Not in the Amygdala." Neuroendocrinology 91.2 (2010): 142-54. Web. 29 Mar. 2015.

16. Sundström-Poromaa, Inger. "Action of Progesterone and Progesterone Metabolites in Menstrual-Cycle–Related Disorders." Headache: The Journal of Head & Face Pain 48 (2008): S90-98. Web. 29 Mar. 2015.

17. Teepker, M., M. Peters, H. Vedder, K. Schepelmann, and S. Lautenbacher. "Menstrual Variation in Experimental Pain: Correlation with Gonadal Hormones." Neuropsychobiology 61.3 (2010): 131-40. Web. 29 Mar. 2015.

18. Turner, Lisa. "Find Hormonal Harmony & Counteract Xenoestrogens Naturally." Better Nutrition 71.5 (2009): 34. Web. 29 Mar. 2015.

19. Zhang, Die, Shen Yang, Chunhao Yang, Guozhang Jin, and Xuechu Zhen. "Estrogen Regulates Responses of Dopamine Neurons in the Ventral Tegmental Area to Cocaine." Psychopharmacology 199.4 (2008): 625-35. Web. 29 Mar. 2015.

20. Zhang, Wanglong, Yu Luo, Li Zhang, Qian Cai, and Xuejun Pan. "Known and Emerging Factors Modulating Estrogenic Effects

of Endocrine-disrupting Chemicals." Environmental Reviews 22.1 (2014): 87-98. Web. 29 Mar. 2015.

21. "Book of All Quotes." Book of All Quotes. N.p., n.d. Web. 13oct.2015, http://www.bookofallquotes.com/

WHY AM I SO TIRED? CHRONIC FATIGUE SYNDROME — MYTH OR REALITY?

1.   Speer L, Mushkbar S. "Doctor, I'm so tired!" Refining your work-up for chronic fatigue. Journal Of Family Practice [serial online]. February 2015;64(2):84-91. Available from: Academic Search Complete, Ipswich, MA. Accessed January 16, 2015.

2.   Teitelbaum J. Effective treatment of chronic fatigue syndrome. Integrative Medicine: A Clinician's Journal [serial online]. December 2011;10(6):44-48. Available from: CINAHL Complete, Ipswich, MA. Accessed January 16, 2015

3.   Teitelbaum J. Chronic fatigue syndrome, fibromyalgia, and myalgic encephalomyelitis: a clinical perspective. Alternative Therapies In Health & Medicine [serial online]. 2014 Jan-Feb 2014;20(1):45-46. Available from: CINAHL Complete, Ipswich, MA. Accessed January 16, 2015

4.   Teitelbaum J. From fatigued to fantastic! Treating CFS, fibromyalgia and myofascial pain. Total Health [serial online]. February 2008;30(1):22-26. Available from: CINAHL Complete, Ipswich, MA. Accessed January 16, 2015

5.   Teitelbaum J, Bird B, Greenfield R, Weiss A, Muenz L, Gould L. Effective treatment of chronic fatigue syndrome and fibromyalgia -- a randomized, double-blind, placebo-controlled, intent-to-treat study. Journal Of Chronic Fatigue Syndrome [serial online]. February 2001;8(2):3-28. Available from: CINAHL Complete, Ipswich, MA. Accessed January 16, 2015

6.   Teitelbaum JE, JA St.Cyr, C Johnson. The use of D-ribose in chronic fatigue syndrome and fibromyalgia: a pilot study. J Alternative and Complementary Medicine 2006;12(9):857-862. http://online.liebertpub.com/doi/abs/10.1089/acm.2006.12.857

7.   Teitelbaum JE, Jandrain J, McGrew R. Effective Treatment of Chronic Fatigue Syndrome and Fibromyalgia with D-ribose—A Multicenter Study. The Open Pain Journal. 2012:5:32-37 http://benthamscience.com/open/topainj/EBM.htm)

8.   Isasi C, Tejerina E, Fernandez-Puga N, Serrano-Vela J. Fibromyalgia and chronic fatigue syndrome caused by non-celiac gluten sensitivity. Reumatología Clínica [serial online]. January 2015;11(1):56-57. Available from: MEDLINE Complete, Ipswich, MA. Accessed January 16, 2015

9.   Jaffe S, Schub T. Chronic Fatigue Syndrome. [serial online]. February 13, 2015;Available from: CINAHL Complete, Ipswich, MA. Accessed January 16, 2015.

10.   CFS case definition. Centers for Disease Control and Prevention Web site. http://

www.cdc.gov/cfs/case-definition/index.html. Revised May 14, 2012. Accessed January 9, 2015

11.   Brown B. Chronic fatigue syndrome: a personalized integrative medicine approach. Alternative Therapies In Health & Medicine [serial online]. 2014 Jan-Feb 2014;20(1):29-40. Available from: CINAHL Complete, Ipswich, MA. Accessed March 16, 2015.

12.   Centers for Disease Control and Prevention. Chronic fatigue syndrome. Centers for Disease Control and Prevention Web site. Available at http://www.cdc.gov/cfs/diagnosis/index.html. Accessed January 6, 2015.

13.   Available at: http://taoofhealing.com/selfcare/ Accessed January 6, 2015.

14. Medical Research on Tai Chi, Qigong/Chronic Fatigue and Immune Dysfunction Syndrome. Available at: http://worldtaichiday.org/medical_research_on_tai_chi_qigong/chronic_fatigue_and_immune_dysfunction_syndrome_cfids.html. Accessed January 6, 2015.

15. "Book of All Quotes." Book of All Quotes. N.p., n.d. Web. 13oct.2015, http://www.bookofallquotes.com/

LET FOOD BE YOUR MEDICINE

1. Becker, Eve. "Watching Your Weight." Living Without 18.2 (2015): 20. Web. 30 Mar. 2015.
2. Bowden, Jonny. "Fat Chances: 10 Surprising and Easy Ways to Get More Healthy Fats in Your Diet." Better Nutrition 74.4 (2012): 44-48. Web. 30 Mar. 2015.
3. Brinkworth, Grant D., Jonathan D. Buckley, Manny Noakes, Peter M. Clifton, and Carlene J. Wilson. "Long-term Effects of a Very Low-Carbohydrate Diet and a Low-Fat Diet on Mood and Cognitive Function." Archives of Internal Medicine 169.20 (2009): 1873-880. Web. 30 Mar. 2015.
4. Brown, Jordana. "Keeping up with Carbing Up." Flex 27.2 (2009): 302. Web. 30 Mar. 2015.
5. Campbell, Amy P., and Tia M. Rains. "Dietary Protein Is Important in the Practical Management of Prediabetes and Type 2 Diabetes." Journal of Nutrition 145.1 (2015): 164S-69S. Web. 30 Mar. 2015.
6. D'Anci, K. E. "Nutrition Updates." Nutrition Reviews. Vol. 68. N.p.: Wiley-Blackwell, 2010. 71-73. Web. 30 Mar. 2015.
7. Dudek, Susan G. Nutrition Essentials for Nursing Practice. Philadelphia: Lippincott Williams & Wilkins, 2010. Print.
8. Filippini, A. "[Low-protein Diet and Nutritional Status]." Giornale Italiano Di Nefrologia: Organo Ufficiale Della Società

Italiana Di Nefrologia 25 Suppl 42 (2008): S39-44. Web. 30 Mar. 2015.

9. Frisoli, Tiberio M., Roland E. Schmieder, Tomasz Grodzicki, and Franz H. Messerli. "Beyond Salt: Lifestyle Modifications and Blood Pressure." European Heart Journal 32.24 (2011): 3081-087. Web. 30 Mar. 2015.

10. Gaesser, Glenn. "Healthy Body, Healthy Mind - Both Fueled by Carbohydrates." Oregon Wheat 65.5 (2013): 22. Web. 30 Mar. 2015.

11. "Getting Your Vitamins and Minerals through Diet. The Benefits of Multivitamins Are Looking Doubtful. Can We Do without Them?" Harvard Women's Health Watch 16.11 (2009): 1-3. Web. 30 Mar. 2015.

12. Gibson, S., P. Gunn, and R., J. Maughan. "Hydration, Water Intake and Beverage Consumption Habits among Adults." Nutrition Bulletin 37.3 (2012): 182-92. Web. 30 Mar. 2015.

13. "High-Protein, Low-Carb, High-Fat Diets May Lower Immune Function." Flex 30.4 (2012): 86. Web. 30 Mar. 2015.

14. Hounsome, N., B. Hounsome, D. Tomos, and G. Edwards-Jones. "Plant Metabolites and Nutritional Quality of Vegetables." Journal of Food Science 73.4 (2008): R48-65. Web. 30 Mar. 2015.

15. Murphy, Suzanne P., Kami K. White, Song-Yi Park, and Sangita Sharma. "Multivitamin-multimineral Supplements' Effect on Total Nutrient Intake." The American Journal Of Clinical Nutrition 85.1 (2007): 280S-84S. Web. 30 Mar. 2015.

16. Raloff, Janet. "Understanding Major Nutrients." Science News for Kids (2008): 3. Web. 30 Mar. 2015.

17. Rietman, Annemarie, Jessica Schwarz, Britt A. Blokker, Els Siebelink, Frans J. Kok, Lydia A. Afman, Daniel Tomé, and Marco Mensink. "Increasing Protein Intake Modulates Lipid Metabolism in Healthy Young Men and Women Consuming a High-fat Hypercaloric Diet." The Journal Of Nutrition 144.8 (2014): 1174-180. Web. 30 Mar. 2015.

18. Sacco, J. E., and V. Tarasuk. "Discretionary Addition of Vitamins and Minerals to Foods: Implications for Healthy Eating." European Journal Of Clinical Nutrition 65.3 (2011): 313-20. Web. 30 Mar. 2015.

19. Slavin, Joanne L., and Beate Lloyd. "Health Benefits of Fruits and Vegetables." Advances In Nutrition (Bethesda, Md.) 3.4 (2012): 506-16. Web. 30 Mar. 2015.

20. Stone, M. "Vegetable Oils Most Suitable for Dietary Consumption." Nutritional Perspectives: Journal of the Council on Nutrition 31.1 (2008): 23-24. Web. 30 Mar. 2015.

21. Sykes, Claire. "Too Much of a Good Thing: Even Healthy Fats Are Best in Moderation." Arthritis Today 26.2 (2012): 23. Web. 30 Mar. 2015.

22. Weisenberger, Jill. "Heart-healthy Fats." Today's Dietitian 15.9 (2013): 14-16. Web. 30 Mar. 2015.

23. Wycherley, T. P., G. D. Brinkworth, J. B. Keogh, M. Noakes, J. D. Buckley, and P. M. Clifton. "Long-term Effects of Weight Loss with a Very Low Carbohydrate and Low Fat Diet on Vascular Function in Overweight and Obese Patients." Journal of Internal Medicine 267.5 (2010): 452-61. Web. 30 Mar. 2015.

24. Zevnik, Neil. "Healing Food. Healthy Vegan: Optimizing Proteins in a Vegan Diet." Better Nutrition 74.4 (2012): 50-54. Web. 30 Mar. 2015.

25. "Book of All Quotes." Book of All Quotes. N.p., n.d. Web. 13oct.2015, http://www.bookofallquotes.com/

WHAT DIET IS BEST FOR YOU?

1. Block, Mary Ann. "Biochemical Individuality Is Important to Women's Health." Business Press 11.9 (1998): 23A. Web. 6 Apr. 2015.

2. Breaux, Theodore A. "Keeping Healthy Balance." American Fitness 28.1 (2010): 66. Web. 6 Apr. 2015.

3.   Chambers, Stephanie, Alexandra Lobb, Laurie T. Butler, and W. Bruce Traill. "The Influence of Age and Gender on Food Choice: A Focus Group Exploration." International Journal of Consumer Studies 32.4 (2008): 356-65. Web. 6 Apr. 2015.

4.   D'Adamo, Peter, and Catherine Whitney. Eat Right 4 (for) Your Type: The Individualized Diet Solution to Staying Healthy, Living Longer & Achieving Your Ideal Weight: 4 Blood Types, 4 Diets. New York: G.P. Putnam's Sons, 1996. Print.

5.   Dudek, Susan G. Nutrition Essentials for Nursing Practice. Philadelphia: Lippincott Williams & Wilkins, 2010. Print.

6.   Ho-Pham, L. T., B. Q. Vu, T. Q. Lai, N. D. Nguyen, and T. V. Nguyen. "Vegetarianism, Bone Loss, Fracture and Vitamin D: A Longitudinal Study in Asian Vegans and Non-vegans." European Journal Of Clinical Nutrition 66.1 (2012): 75-82. Web. 6 Apr. 2015.

7.   Lagiou, Pagona, Sven Sandin, Marie Lof, Dimitrios Trichopoulos, Hans-Olov Adami, and Elisabete Weiderpass. "Low Carbohydrate-high Protein Diet and Incidence of Cardiovascular Diseases in Swedish Women: Prospective Cohort Study." BMJ: British Medical Journal (Overseas & Retired Doctors Edition) 345.7864 (2012): 14. Web. 6 Apr. 2015.

8.   Neustadt, J., and S. Pieczenik. "Biochemical Individuality." Integrative Medicine: A Clinician's Journal 6.3 (2007): 30-32. Web. 6 Apr. 2015.

9.   Orlich, Michael J., Pramil N. Singh, Joan Sabaté, Karen Jaceldo-Siegl, Jing Fan, Synnove Knutsen, W. Lawrence Beeson, and Gary E. Fraser. "Vegetarian Dietary Patterns and Mortality in Adventist Health Study 2." JAMA Internal Medicine 173.13 (2013): 1230-238. Web. 6 Apr. 2015.

10.   Pawlak, Roman, Scott James Parrott, Sudha Raj, Diana Cullum-Dugan, and Debbie Lucus. "How Prevalent Is Vitamin B(12) Deficiency among Vegetarians?" Nutrition Reviews 71.2 (2013): 110-17. Web. 6 Apr. 2015.

11. Pilis, Wiesław, Krzysztof Stec, Michał Zych, and Anna Pilis. "Health Benefits and Risk Associated with Adopting a Vegetarian Diet." Roczniki Państwowego Zakładu Higieny 65.1 (2014): 9-14. Web. 6 Apr. 2015.

12. Rosenthal, Joshua. Integrative Nutrition: Feed Your Hunger for Health and Happiness. New York, NY: Integrative Nutrition Pub., 2008. Print.

13. Wardle, Jane, Anne M. Haase, Andrew Steptoe, Maream Nillapun, Kiriboon Jonwutiwes, and France Bellisle. "Gender Differences in Food Choice: The Contribution of Health Beliefs and Dieting." Annals of Behavioral Medicine 27.2 (2004): 107-16. Web. 6 Apr. 2015.

14. "Book of All Quotes." Book of All Quotes. N.p., n.d. Web. 13oct.2015, http://www.bookofallquotes.com/

HEALING POWER OF SLEEP

1. Tweed J. The healing power of a good night's sleep. Lake Country Journal. 2012; 51-52.

2. Saper CB, Scammell TE, Lu J. Hypothalamic regulation of sleep and circadian rhythms. Nature. 2005; 437: 1257-1263. doi:10.1038/nature04284.

3. Oxtoby K. Sleepless nights: The role you can play in tackling insomnia. Chemist & Druggist. 2012; 23-25.

4. medicalnewstoday.com/articles/249592.php

5. "CircadianRhythms."Nigms.nih.gov. N.p., n.d. Web 13Oct.2015'http://www.nigms.nih.gov/Education/Pages/Factsheet_CircadianRhythms.aspx

6. "Book of All Quotes." Book of All Quotes. N.p., n.d. Web. 13oct.2015, http://www.bookofallquotes.com/

HEALING POWER OF MOVEMENT

1. Wells C, Kolt GS, Marshall P, Hill B, Bialocerkowski A. The Effectiveness of Pilates Exercise in People with Chronic Low Back Pain: A Systematic Review. PLoS ONE. 2014; 9(7): e100402. doi:10.1371/journal.pone.0100402.

2. Wentworth A. Helping Patients Discover the Benefits of Exercise. Coming of Age. 2014; 7-10.

3. Teo W, Newton M J, McGuigan MR. Circadian rhythms in exercise performance: Implications for hormonal and muscular adaptation. Journal of Sports Science and Medicine. 2011; 10: 600-606.

4. Wren P. Weight Training for Women. Alive. 2014; 61-65.

5. Grote D. Are You Over-exercising? Washingtonian Magazine. 2014; 109-112.

6. Foston M. 4 Steps to a Safe Workout. Alive. 2014; 112-115.

7. Matusek J. HIIT Yourself Up. Ultimate MMA. 2013; 70.

8. Roxburgh BH, Nolan PB, Weatherwax RM, Dalleck LC. Is Moderate Intensity Exercise Training Combined with High Intensity Interval Training More Effective at Improving Cardiorespiratory Fitness than Moderate Intensity Exercise Training Alone? Journal of Sports Science and Medicine. 2014; 13: 702-707.

9. Smith JA, Greer T, Sheets T, Watson S. Is There More to Yoga Than Exercise? Alternative Therapies. 2011; 13(3): 22-29.

10. Ross A. The Health Benefits of Yoga and Exercise: A Review of Comparison Studies. The Journal of Alternative and Complementary Medicine. 2010; (16 1): 3–12. doi: 10.1089=acm.2009.0044.

11. "Book of All Quotes." Book of All Quotes. N.p., n.d. Web. 13oct.2015, http://www.bookofallquotes.com/

BEAUTIFUL YOU

1.   Almeida, Jose I., and Jeffrey K. Raines. "Laser Ablation of Cutaneous Leg Veins." *Perspectives In Vascular Surgery And Endovascular Therapy* 20.4 (2008): 358-66. Web. 10 Apr. 2015.

2.   Betsi, Evelyn-Evanthia, Esnault Germain, Daniel Kalbermatten, Mathias Tremp, and Veronique Emmenegger. "Platelet-rich Plasma Injection Is Effective and Safe for the Treatment of Alopecia." *European Journal of Plastic Surgery* 36.7 (2013): 407-12. Web. 10 Apr. 2015.

3.   Cervelli, V., S. Garcovich, A. Bielli, G. Cervelli, B. C. Curcio, M. G. Scioli, A. Orlandi, and P. Gentile. "The Effect of Autologous Activated Platelet Rich Plasma (AA-PRP) Injection on Pattern Hair Loss: Clinical and Histomorphometric Evaluation." *Biomed Research International* 2014 (2014): 760709. Web. 10 Apr. 2015.

4.   Colino, Stacey. "Timeless BEAUTY." *Natural Health* 36.3 (2006): 78. Web. 10 Apr. 2015.

5.   El-Azhary, Rokea A., and Jolleen A. Weick. "Sclerotherapy of Spider Veins Using the Accurate Depth-gauge Collagen Needle." *International Journal Of Dermatology* 47.2 (2008): 205-06. Web. 10 Apr. 2015.

6.   Fernandez, Alexandra A., Katlein França, Anna H. Chacon, and Keyvan Nouri. "From Flint Razors to Lasers: A Timeline of Hair Removal Methods." *Journal of Cosmetic Dermatology* 12.2 (2013): 153-62. Web. 10 Apr. 2015.

7.   Grunewald, Sonja, Marc Oliver Bodendorf, Alexander Zygouris, Jan Christoph Simon, and Uwe Paasch. "Long-term Efficacy of Linear-scanning 808 Nm Diode Laser for Hair Removal Compared to a Scanned Alexandrite Laser." *Lasers In Surgery And Medicine* 46.1 (2014): 13-19. Web. 10 Apr. 2015.

8.   Khunger, Niti, and S. Sacchidanand. "Standard Guidelines for Care: Sclerotherapy in Dermatology." *Indian Journal of Dermatology, Venereology & Leprology* 77.2 (2011): 222-31. Web. 10 Apr. 2015.

9.   Landau, Marina. "Combination of Chemical Peelings with Botulinum Toxin Injections and Dermal Fillers." *Journal of Cosmetic Dermatology* 5.2 (2006): 121-26. Web. 10 Apr. 2015.

10.   Letessier, S. "Treatment of Wrinkles with Botulinum Toxin." *Journal of Dermatological Treatment* 10.1 (1999): 31. Web. 10 Apr. 2015.

11.   Lipozenčić, Jasna, and Zrinka Bukvić Mokos. "Dermatologic Lasers in the Treatment of Aging Skin." *Acta Dermatovenerologica Croatica: ADC* 18.3 (2010): 176-80. Web. 10 Apr. 2015.

12.   Moreno-Moraga, Javier, Josefina Royo, Adriana Smarandache, Mihail L. Pascu, and Mario A. Trelles. "1064 Nm Nd:YAG Long Pulse Laser after Polidocanol Microfoam Injection Dramatically Improves the Result of Leg Vein Treatment: A Randomized Controlled Trial on 517 Legs with a Three-year Follow-up." *Phlebology* 29.10 (2014): 658-66. Web. 10 Apr. 2015.

13.   Ogden, S., and T.W. Griffiths. "A Review of Minimally Invasive Cosmetic Procedures." *British Journal of Dermatology* 159.5 (2008): 1036-050. Web. 10 Apr. 2015.

14.   O'mahony, Malti. "Microdermabrasion: Indications, Devices, Treatment Protocols and Clinic Data." *Journal of Aesthetic Nursing* 3.9 (2014): 430-35. Web. 10 Apr. 2015.

15.   Rao, Krishna, and Thangasamy K. Sankar. "Long-pulsed Nd:YAG Laser-assisted Hair Removal in Fitzpatrick Skin Types IV-VI." *Lasers In Medical Science* 26.5 (2011): 623-26. Web. 10 Apr. 2015.

16.   Rendon, Marta I., Diane S. Berson, Joel L. Cohen, Wendy E. Roberts, Isaac Starker, and Beatrice Wang. "Evidence and Considerations in the Application of Chemical Peels in Skin Disorders and Aesthetic Resurfacing."*Journal of Clinical & Aesthetic Dermatology* 3.7 (2010): 32-43. Web. 10 Apr. 2015.

17.   Singal, Archana, Sidharth Sonthalia, and Prashant Verma. "Female Pattern Hair Loss." *Indian Journal of Dermatology, Venereology & Leprology* 79.5 (2013): 626-40. Web. 10 Apr. 2015.

18. Tran, Diana, Joshua P. Townley, Tanya M. Barnes, and Kerryn A. Greive. "An Antiaging Skin Care System Containing Alpha Hydroxy Acids and Vitamins Improves the Biomechanical Parameters of Facial Skin."*Clinical, Cosmetic And Investigational Dermatology* 8 (2014): 9-17. Web. 10 Apr. 2015.

19. Turlier, Virginie, Amandine Rouquier, David Black, Gwendal Josse, Arielle Auvergnat, Alain Briant, Serge Dahan, Véronique Gassia, Christine Saint-Martory, Wassim Zakaria, Catherine Queille-Roussel, Catherine Grognard-Gourdon, Daphné Thioly-Bensoussan, Arnaud Degouy, and Anne-Marie Schmitt. "Assessment of the Clinical Efficacy of a Hyaluronic Acid-based Deep Wrinkle Filler Using New Instrumental Methods."*Journal of Cosmetic & Laser Therapy* 12.4 (2010): 195-202. Web. 10 Apr. 2015.

20. Van Zuuren, E. J., Z. Fedorowicz, and B. Carter. "Evidence-based Treatments for Female Pattern Hair Loss: A Summary of a Cochrane Systematic Review." *The British Journal Of Dermatology* 167.5 (2012): 995-1010. Web. 10 Apr. 2015.

21. Vedamurthy, Maya. "Standard Guidelines for the Use of Dermal Fillers." *Indian Journal of Dermatology, Venereology & Leprology* (2008): S23-27. Web. 10 Apr. 2015.

22. "Women Can Win the Fight Against Common Forms of Hair Loss." *Dermatology Nursing* 22.5 (2010): 39-40. Web. 10 Apr. 2015.

23. ."Book of All Quotes." Book of All Quotes. N.p., n.d. Web. 13oct.2015, http://www.bookofallquotes.com/

24. "Understanding UVA and UVB." Skincancer.N.p.,n.d.Web.15 Oct. 2015<www.skincancer.org>

25. "Physical vs Chemical Sunscreens" Skinacea N.p.,n.d.Web.15 Oct. 2015http://www.skinacea.com/.

26. "Skin Types vs Skin Conditions." Dermascope Magazine. Web.15 Oct. 2015http://www.dermascope.com/.

PART III — HEALING THE SOUL

1.   Amen, Daniel G. *Healing the Hardware of the Soul: Enhance Your Brain to Improve Your Work, Love, and Spiritual Life.* United States of America: Free, 2008. *Book Review Digest Plus (H.W. Wilson).* Web. 28 Nov. 2015.

2.   Amen, Daniel G. *Sex on the Brain: 12 Lessons to Enhance Your Love Life.* United States of America: Harmony, 2007. *Book Review Digest Plus (H.W. Wilson).* Web. 28 Nov. 2015.

3.   Amen, Daniel G. "Unleash The Power Of The Female Brain...Daniel G Amen, MD." *Life Extension* (2014): 1-3 3p. *Ccm.* Web. 28 Nov. 2015.

4.   "Bestseller Stat Shot." *Publishers Weekly* 262.30 (2015): 2. *Business Source Complete.* Web. 28 Nov. 2015.

5.   Bitzer, Johannes, Annamaria Giraldi, and Jim Pfaus. "Sexual Desire and Hypoactive Sexual Desire Disorder in Women. Introduction and Overview. Standard Operating Procedure (SOP Part 1)." *The Journal Of Sexual Medicine* 10.1 (2013): 36-49. *MEDLINE Complete.* Web. 28 Nov. 2015.

6.   Brandon, Marianne, and Andrew Goldstein. *Reclaiming Desire: 4 Keys to Finding Your Lost Libido.* United States of America: Rodale, 2004. *Book Review Digest Plus (H.W. Wilson).* Web. 28 Nov. 2015.

7.   Brotto, Lori A., A. John Petkau, Fernand Labrie, and Rosemary Basson. "Predictors of Sexual Desire Disorders in Women." *The Journal Of Sexual Medicine* 8.3 (2011): 742-53. *MEDLINE Complete.* Web. 28 Nov. 2015.

8.   Burrows, Lara J., Maureen Basha, and Andrew T. Goldstein. "The Effects of Hormonal Contraceptives on Female Sexuality: A Review." *The Journal Of Sexual Medicine* 9.9 (2012): 2213-223. *MEDLINE Complete.* Web. 28 Nov. 2015.

9.   Chopra, Deepak. "Secret of Love." *Personal Excellence Essentials* 18.4 (2013): 16. *Business Source Complete.* Web. 28 Nov. 2015.

10. Chopra, Deepak. "The Self-esteem Repair Kit." *Australian Women's Weekly* 78.7 (2008): 116. *MasterFILE Complete*. Web. 28 Nov. 2015.

11. Chopra, Deepak. "Who Am I?" *International Professional Performance Magazine* 16.3 (2008): 14. *Business Source Complete*. Web. 28 Nov. 2015.

12. Del Corso, Annalisa Rossi, and Margherita Lanz. "Felt Obligation and the Family Life Cycle: A Study on Intergenerational Relationships." *International Journal of Psychology* 48.6 (2013): 1196-200. *PsycINFO*. Web. 28 Nov. 2015.

13. Ekholm, Ulla-Britt, Sahruh Turkmen, Stefan Hammarbäck, and Torbjörn Bäckström. "Sexuality and Androgens in Women with Cyclical Mood Changes and Pre-menstrual Syndrome." *Acta Obstetricia Et Gynecologica Scandinavica* 93.3 (2014): 248-55. *MEDLINE Complete*. Web. 28 Nov. 2015.

14. "Fifty Shades: By the Numbers." *Publishers Weekly* 262.23 (2015): 14. *Business Source Complete*. Web. 28 Nov. 2015.

15. Goulston, Mark. *Just Listen: Discover the Secret to Getting through to Absolutely Anyone*. N.p.: American Management Association, 2009. *Book Review Digest Plus (H.W. Wilson)*. Web. 28 Nov. 2015.

16. Hall, Kathryn. *Reclaiming Your Sexual Self: How You Can Bring Desire Back into Your Life*. United States of America: John Wiley & Sons, 2004. *Book Review Digest Plus (H.W. Wilson)*. Web. 28 Nov. 2015.

17. Heiman, Julia R., Heather Rupp, Erick Janssen, Sarah K. Newhouse, Marieke Brauer, and Ellen Laan. "Sexual Desire, Sexual Arousal and Hormonal Differences in Premenopausal US and Dutch Women with and without Low Sexual Desire." *Hormones And Behavior* 59.5 (2011): 772-79. *MEDLINE Complete*. Web. 28 Nov. 2015.

18. Jung, Carl Gustav. *The Integration of the Personality*. N.p.: Farrar, 1939. *Brr*. Web. 28 Nov. 2015.

19. Kalmbach, David A., and Vivek Pillai. "Daily Affect and Female Sexual Function." *The Journal Of Sexual Medicine* 11.12 (2014): 2938-954. *MEDLINE Complete*. Web. 28 Nov. 2015.

20. Letessier, S. "Treatment of Wrinkles with Botulinum Toxin." *Journal of Dermatological Treatment* 10.1 (1999): 31. *Academic Search Complete*. Web. 28 Nov. 2015.

21. Mcmillan, Ron, Kerry Patterson, Joseph Grenny, and Al Switzler. *Crucial Conversations: Tools for Talking When Stakes Are High*. United States of America: McGraw-Hill, 2011. *Book Review Digest Plus (H.W. Wilson)*. Web. 28 Nov. 2015.

22. Nichols, Michael P. *The Lost Art of Listening: How Learning to Listen Can Improve Relationships*. United States of America: Guilford, 1995. *Book Review Digest Plus (H.W. Wilson)*. Web. 28 Nov. 2015.

23. Nishimoto, Patricia, and Una Starr. "Supporting the Couple With Female Dyspareunia." *Clinical Journal Of Oncology Nursing* 19.4 (2015): 390-92. *MEDLINE Complete*. Web. 28 Nov. 2015.

24. Reviriego, C. "Flibanserin for Female Sexual Dysfunction." *Drugs Of Today (Barcelona, Spain: 1998)* 50.8 (2014): 549-56. *MEDLINE Complete*. Web. 28 Nov. 2015.

25. Roos, Anne-Marie, Ranee Thakar, Abdul H. Sultan, Curt W. Burger, and Aggie T G Paulus. "Pelvic Floor Dysfunction: Women's Sexual Concerns Unraveled." *The Journal Of Sexual Medicine* 11.3 (2014): 743-52. *MEDLINE Complete*. Web. 28 Nov. 2015.

26. Simon, James A., Rossella E. Nappi, Sheryl A. Kingsberg, Ricardo Maamari, and Vivien Brown. "Clarifying Vaginal Atrophy's Impact on Sex and Relationships (CLOSER) Survey: Emotional and Physical Impact of Vaginal Discomfort on North American Postmenopausal Women and Their Partners." *Menopause (10723714)* 21.2 (2014): 137-42 6p. *Ccm*. Web. 28 Nov. 2015.

27. Sprecher, Susan, James E. Brooks, and Winfred Avogo. "Self-esteem among Young Adults: Differences and Similarities Based on Gender, Race, and Cohort (1990–2012)." *Sex Roles* 69.5-6 (2013): 264-75. *PsycINFO*. Web. 28 Nov. 2015.

28. Van Anders, Sari M. "Testosterone and Sexual Desire in Healthy Women and Men." *Archives Of Sexual Behavior* 41.6 (2012): 1471-484. *MEDLINE Complete*. Web. 28 Nov. 2015.

29. Versey, H. Shellae. "Managing Work and Family: Do Control Strategies Help?" *Developmental Psychology* 51.11 (2015): 1672-681. *PsycINFO*. Web. 28 Nov. 2015.

30. Wåhlin-Jacobsen, Sarah, Anette Tønnes Pedersen, Ellids Kristensen, Nanna Cassandra Laessøe, Marika Lundqvist, Arieh S. Cohen, David M. Hougaard, and Annamaria Giraldi. "Is There a Correlation between Androgens and Sexual Desire in Women?" *The Journal Of Sexual Medicine* 12.2 (2015): 358-73. *MEDLINE Complete*. Web. 28 Nov. 2015.

31. "Book of All Quotes." Book of All Quotes. N.p., n.d. Web. 13oct.2015, http://www.bookofallquotes.com/

PART IV— SELF TRANSFORMATION

1. "Beauty 101." *Good Health (Australia Edition)* (2010): 134. *MasterFILE Complete*. Web. 28 Nov. 2015.

2. Bengtson, Bradley P., and Caroline A. Glicksman. "The Standardization of Bra Cup Measurements: Redefining Bra Sizing Language." *Clinics In Plastic Surgery* 42.4 (2015): 405-11. *MEDLINE Complete*. Web. 28 Nov. 2015.

3. Durning, Marijke Vroomen. "Fitting Your Bra." *Alive* 369 (2013): 81. *MasterFILE Complete*. Web. 28 Nov. 2015.

4. Furusawa, Masahiro, Jun-ichi Takahashi, Motoko Isoyama, Yoshiko Kitamura, Tomoko Kashima, Fumie Ueshima, Noriko Nakahama, Misako Araki, Yasuko Rokukawa, Yoshikazu Takahashi, Takemi Makiishi, and Ken-ichi Yatabe. "Effectiveness of Dental Checkups Incorporating Tooth Brushing Instruction." *The Bulletin Of Tokyo Dental College* 52.3 (2011): 129-33. *MEDLINE Complete*. Web. 28 Nov. 2015.

5. "Is Exercise Really Medicine? The Many Benefits of Physical Activity Are Continually Backed by Mounting Research." *Harvard Health Letter / From Harvard Medical School* 39.10 (2014): 1. *MEDLINE Complete*. Web. 28 Nov. 2015.

6.   Kokkinos, Peter. "Physical Activity, Health Benefits, And Mortality Risk." *ISRN Cardiology* (2012): 1-14 14p. *Ccm.* Web. 28 Nov. 2015.

7.   Lange, Rose M. "Physical Activity Levels in Obese and Non-obese Women and Their Relationship with Body Mass Index, Perceived Self-efficacy, Perceived Benefits and Barriers of Exercise, and Commitment to a Plan of Action." Thesis. Pro Quest Information & Learning, n.d. *Dissertation Abstracts International: Section B: The Sciences and Engineering* 71.7-B (2011): 4173. *PsycINFO.* Web. 28 Nov. 2015.

8.   "Make the Most of Your Shape." *Marie Claire (US Edition)* 13.3 (2006): 189. *MasterFILE Complete.* Web. 28 Nov. 2015.

9.   Meisel, Steve. "The Body Eclectic." *Vogue* 192.4 (2002): 162. *MasterFILE Complete.* Web. 28 Nov. 2015.

10.   Miyabara, Y., D. Holmes, J. Camp, V. M. Miller, and A. E. Kearns. "Comparison of Calibrated and Uncalibrated Bone Mineral Density by CT to DEXA in Menopausal Women." *Climacteric* 15.4 (2012): 374-81. *Academic Search Complete.* Web. 28 Nov. 2015.

11.   "Nashville Boot Camp Owner: Even a Little Cardio Exercise Can Go a Long Way." *Tennessee Tribune* 22.32 (2011): 3A. *MasterFILE Complete.* Web. 28 Nov. 2015.

12.   Oeffinger, Kevin C., Elizabeth T. H. Fontham, Ruth Etzioni, Abbe Herzig, James S. Michaelson, Ya-Chen Tina Shih, Louise C. Walter, Timothy R. Church, Christopher R. Flowers, Samuel J. Lamonte, Andrew M. D. Wolf, Carol Desantis, Joannie Lortet-Tieulent, Kimberly Andrews, Deana Manassaram-Baptiste, Debbie Saslow, Robert A. Smith, Otis W. Brawley, and Richard Wender. "Breast Cancer Screening for Women at Average Risk: 2015 Guideline Update From the American Cancer Society." *JAMA: Journal of the American Medical Association* 314.15 (2015): 1599-614 16p. *Ccm.* Web. 28 Nov. 2015.

13.   Pai, Deanna. "Playing the Skin-Care Field?" *Cosmopolitan* 259.2 (2015): 98. *MasterFILE Complete.* Web. 28 Nov. 2015.

14. Qaseem, Amir, Thomas D. Denberg, Robert H. Hopkins Jr., Linda L. Humphrey, Joel Levine, Donna E. Sweet, and Paul Shekelle. "Screening for Colorectal Cancer: A Guidance Statement From the American College of Physicians." *Annals of Internal Medicine* 156.5 (2012): 378-W-114. *Academic Search Complete*. Web. 28 Nov. 2015.

15. Rados, Carol. "Science Meets Beauty: Using Medicine to Improve Appearances." *FDA Consumer* 38.2 (2004): 30-35. *General Science Full Text (H.W. Wilson)*. Web. 28 Nov. 2015.

16. Stevens, Sidney, and Ronald L. Hoffman. *How to Talk with Your Doctor: The Guide for Patients and Their Physicians Who Want to Reconcile and Use the Best of Conventional and Alternative Medicine*. N.p.: Basic Health Publications, 2006.

17. Thomas, Pat. *Ecologist* 36.5 (2006): 062-63. *Hus*. Web.

18. "Why You Need a Bone Density Scan." *Harvard Women's Health Watch* 21.7 (2014): 3-3 1p. *Ccm*. Web. 28 Nov. 2015.

19. www.cancer.gov

20. www.cdc.gov

21. "Book of All Quotes." Book of All Quotes. N.p., n.d. Web. 13oct.2015, http://www.bookofallquotes.com/

ABOUT THE AUTHOR

Natalya Fazylova is a Doctor of Nursing Practice and an Associate Professor at the City University of New York. In her postgraduate education Dr. Fazylova became a certified Chinese Herbologist through the New York Institute of Herbal Medicine and a Certified Integrative Nutrition Health Coach through the Institute of Integrative Nutrition. She is ANCC Board Certified in Adult Health, as a Holistic Health Practitioner by the American Association of Drugless Practitioners and Board Certified as an Integrative Medicine Practitioner by The American Association of Integrative Medicine.

Dr. Fazylova earned her Bachelor and Master of Science from Hunter Bellevue School of Nursing and her Doctor of Nursing Practice from PACE University. Her doctorate work on topic of "Reduction of Childhood Obesity via the Web-Based Programs in School-Aged Children" was presented at the Sigma Theta Tau International Research Conference in Hong Kong. She is a recipient of Patricia McGee Nursing Faculty Scholarship Award and a Finalist in the Nursing Spectrum Excellence Awards for Clinical Care. Dr. Fazylova was included in the 2010-2011 Edition of Sutton Who's Who in Academia and Cambridge Who's Who Registry among Executives and Professionals in the field of Research, Medicine and Health Care. She serves as a writer and editor of a health section column in a Russian American Magazine "World Voice". Dr. Fazylova is a member of the Sigma Theta Tau International Honor Society, American Academy of Anti -Aging Medicine and American Association of Integrative Medicine.

Dr. Fazylova's passion is to provide a holistic and integrative care bringing healing modalities from both Eastern and Western Medicine in her practice.

Made in the USA
Middletown, DE
21 March 2017